Biomedical Statistics
with Computing

MEDICAL COMPUTING SERIES

Series Editor: **Dr. D. W. Hill**
North East Thames Regional Health Authority, London, England

1. Computers in Ultrasonic Diagnostics
   P. N. T. Wells *and* **John P. Woodcock**

2. Computers for the Physician's Office
   Joan Zimmerman *and* **Alan Rector**

3. Mathematical Modelling of Dynamic Biological Systems
   Ludwik Finkelstein *and* **Ewart R. Carson**

4. Techniques for the Analysis and Modelling of Enzyme Kinetic Mechanisms
   Chan F. Lam

5. Computers in Radiotherapy Planning
   Raymond G. Wood

6. Biomedical Statistics with Computing
   Mary H. Regier, Ram N. Mohapatra *and* **Surya N. Mohapatra**

Biomedical Statistics with Computing

Mary H. Regier, Ph.D.,
Ram N. Mohapatra, Ph.D.
Professors of Statistics and Mathematics,
American University of Beirut, Lebanon

and

Surya N. Mohapatra, Ph.D.
Nuclear Magnetic Resonance Imaging, Picker International, and
Research Department of Anaesthetics, Royal College of
Surgeons of England

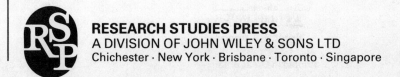

RESEARCH STUDIES PRESS
A DIVISION OF JOHN WILEY & SONS LTD
Chichester · New York · Brisbane · Toronto · Singapore

RESEARCH STUDIES PRESS

Editorial Office:
58B Station Road, Letchworth, Herts. SG6 3BE, England

British Library Cataloguing in Publication Data:

Regier, Mary H.
    Biomedical statistics with computing.—(Medical
    computing series)
    1. Medical statistics
    I. Title   II. Mohapatra, Surya N.
    III. Mohapatra, Ram N.   IV. Series
    519.5'02461   RA409

    ISBN 0 471 10449 3

Typesetting and layout by
    —les éditions———
    L'Orient-LE JOUR
                     S A L

    Beirut — Lebanon

Printed in Great Britain

To: Frank, Terry and Chris
M.H.R.

To: Jhunu, Raju, Seema and Manas
R.N.M.

To: Valli and Rahul
S.N.M.

Preface

This book is intended to serve both as an introduction to the basic statistical methods and as a practical guide in their application. Although it addresses itself to the biomedical scientist, with data in the illustrative examples originating mainly in biological and medical experiments, the presentation is quite general, and the user from any other discipline can equally well adapt the methods to his own needs.

The mathematical prerequisites for the use of this book are minimal and do not go beyond the usual high school level, with no previous knowledge of statistics or of computer languages assumed. Beginning with the relatively elementary techniques of descriptive statistics, the various statistical methods are presented with emphasis on their logic and utility rather than through mathematical derivations. Our computer programs are written in CP/M BASIC and run on a Pertec PCC 2000. Users with access to any desk-top computer need only acquaint themselves with the special features of that computer and the particular form of BASIC appropriate to it; a few changes in the commands may be necessary before the package of programs is used.

The book is intended for use by several types of readers. The scientist who wishes to become acquainted with the commonly used statistical methods without taking a formal course in the subject may find a systematic reading of the chapters a convenient way to do so. Other readers may wish to use the book as a reference, and for this purpose the chapters are organized as units, each dealing with a particular problem and covering as many aspects of the problem as was considered possible in a book of this size. To facilitate the computations that usually accompany any statistical analysis, we have provided a package of computer programs that may be stored on disc for repeated applications of the method to different sets of data. The programs are grouped in the last chapter, with cross-references between each program and the other pages on which the methods are described and commented upon. Each program is self-contained, however, and is illustrated with data that appeared in a previous chapter, where computations were carried out with the use of a calculator. The entire package of programs is preceded by a brief introduction to the computer language BASIC, including definitions of some of its frequently used commands.

The book may also be used as a textbook for an introductory course in statistical methods for students in the biological and medical sciences. For such use, it is expected that the instructor will provide data which would serve as exercises in the course and which would come from investigations of 'interest to the class. The data that was used in many of the illustrative examples in the book were supplied to the authors by the original investigators.

The authors wish to thank all their colleagues who have so generously contributed their data as well as those who have assisted in the collection of data. Thanks are also due to authors who have given permission for the use of their previously published data. We are grateful to the RAND Corporation for permission to reproduce page 363 from *A Million Random Digits with 100,000 Normal Deviates* and to the Biometrika Trustees for permission to reproduce material from *Biometrika Tables for Statisticians,* Vol. 1 (3rd edition, 1966), Tables 8, 18, 12, 22 and 27. We are also grateful to the Literary Executor of the late Sir Ronald A. Fisher, F.R.S., to Dr. Frank Yates, F.R.S., and to Longman Group Ltd. London, for permission to reprint Table II 1, page 45, from their book *Statistical Tables for Biological, Agricultural and Medical Research* (6th edition, 1974).

A grant to the first author from the Arts and Sciences Research Fund, American University of Beirut, was of great help in covering expenses connected with the preparation of the manuscript, and is hereby gratefully acknowledged.

The authors also wish to express their gratitude to Dr. D. W. Hill, editor of this series, for his interest and encouragement.

Beirut, Lebanon   M.H.R.
March 1982   R.N.M.
                                         S.N.M.

Table of Contents

CHAPTER 1
Introduction

Statistics has long been recognized as a valuable tool in the analysis of biomedical data, and the constant refinements and innovations in statistical techniques have usually found receptive ground for application in the health and medical sciences. In recent years, this interest in statistics has become increasingly widespread. A growing number of research scientists and clinicians are now relying on standard statistical routines for the planning of data collection and the analysis of their observations. The general availability of calculators and computers, and the resulting reduction in computational chores, have undoubtedly encouraged and accelerated this trend.

Examples of the many ways in which statistical methods are being utilized to great advantage in the service of medical and related studies can be found in most of the professional journals. A large number of examples also appear in the following chapters in connection with the various concepts and methods that are presented. These examples serve both as numerical illustrations for the methods and as a guide in the interpretation of computational results. Although they are drawn almost exclusively from the biological and medical sciences, they should equally be of interest to the reader from any other discipline.

The book presupposes no special knowledge of statistics; neither are computer facilities essential for its use. Yet it is hoped that even readers who are familiar with all the methods covered in the book will find certain aspects of it useful for their purposes. Both the selection and organization of material have been motivated by a desire to serve the needs of users at various levels of familiarity with the subject and with different computing facilities at their disposal.

For the reader with no previous training in the use of statistical methods, it is recommended that the chapters be read through carefully and in the given sequence. It is also recommended that the calculations in the examples be verified wherever possible and, if a microcomputer is to be used, that the corresponding programs be applied to the same data and output checked against results given in the illustrations.

Readers who are familiar with the methods and only need easy references for specific tasks can turn to the chapter that deals with the particular problem. The organization into chapters by type of problem rather than by method will be found a convenience since, in addition to a description of the appropriate techniques and specification of conditions for their use, each chapter contains illustrations and comments that might prove useful in the analysis. Of particular importance is the statement of assumptions under which certain methods are applicable to the observations. A routine application of a method to a given set of data may very well lead to erroneous conclusions if the data does not satisfy the assumptions on which the method is based.

The book is also addressed to those readers who wish to have at their disposal a package of statistical programs that can be used in conjunction with a desk-top microcomputer. Such a self-contained unit of programs is given in Chapter 18 and can be used independently of the rest of the book by anyone who is fully acquainted with the background, motivations, assumptions and interpretations of the various statistical methods. For the benefit of other users of the package, references are made in each of its units to those sections in previous chapters that deal with the method, so that the necessary details for its implementation can be easily filled in.

As with any book of this nature, a certain amount of groundwork and definitions of terms have to precede the outlining of procedures. These preliminaries are given in the next four chapters. In Chapter 2, we define populations and samples and describe data collecting as the process of making repeated observations on variables in a population. The various types of variables are defined in Chapter 3, and appropriate ways for handling data of the different types are presented. These include ways of organizing the observations and making tabular or graphical summaries which are often useful in the subsequent analysis. Chapter 4 contains an introduction to probability, some typical probability distributions, and a definition of quantities with which the methods of later chapters are concerned. The two basic methods of classical statistical inference, interval estimation and hypothesis testing, are introduced in Chapter 5 without reference to any particular application. Their applications to specific problems, which depend in each case on the type of variable as well as on the aim of the investigation, are outlined in Chapters 6 through 16. A few typical pitfalls in the applications of statistical methods are described and commented on in Chapter 17. Chapter 18 contains 27 programs for optional use in the computational part of the analysis.

The packaged programs of Chapter 18 are written in CP/M BASIC. They are readily adaptable for use on any microcomputer and may be stored on a memory disc for repeated applications as the need arises. However, if a microcomputer is not easily accessible, this is not a serious shortcoming, as most of the calculations called for in the methods can be carried out on a relatively simple pocket calculator. Some calculators come equipped with special statistical function keys, which considerably reduce the computational labor, while more elaborate ones may be programmed with one's selection of frequently used formulas. The one method that requires computational facilities more sophisticated than the ones mentioned thus far is the analysis of multiple regression discussed in Section 14.8. Once a formidable computational task, multiple regression can now be easily carried out with the help of one of many statistical packages available for use on a high speed digital computer. Packages such as SPSS, BMDP, and others have been standard software at computer centers for many years and are periodically updated, while new ones are being developed both for general and specific purposes. The investigator should have no difficulty in finding a package to suit his needs. Indeed, some may find it convenient to use such a package for the less complex statistical calculations as well.

The statistical techniques incorporated into packaged programs and all those outlined in the following chapters consist of well-established routines that are commonly applied in standard statistical analysis. While this is sufficient for most of the needs of the biomedical scientist, situations arise from time to time that call for approaches of a non-routine nature. In cases like these, a statistician is usually consulted, and some modifications are made in the standard procedure, or an entirely new procedure is worked out, so that the problem could conceivably lead to fresh developments in statistical methodology. It is in response to challenges of this nature in the various sciences that new statistical methods and techniques have evolved over the years. In particular, statistics owes a great deal of its growth to the impetus provided by quantitative problems in biological and medical studies, and the benefits it shares with these sciences are thus reciprocal.

CHAPTER 2
Collection of Data

2.1. POPULATIONS AND SAMPLES

Statistical methods are techniques applied to sets of observations on well-defined groups of elements. The observed characteristic is called the *variable*, and the set of all possible observations on this variable is called the *population*. As can be seen in the following examples, the variable may be numerical or qualitative, single or composite, depending upon the type of information sought by the experimenter.

Example 2.1. Suppose we are interested in the ages of patients in a particular hospital on a given day. The characteristic to be observed here is age, a numerical variable, and the ages of all the patients, being the set of all possible observations, is the population.

Example 2.2. Suppose that there are 750 workers in a certain factory and that we wish to investigate their blood types. The variable, blood type, is a qualitative variable, and the set of all 750 blood types, each corresponding to one of the workers, constitutes the population.

Example 2.3. In a feeding experiment, we wish to study the effect of a special diet on the weights of the N guinea pigs in our laboratory. Let X denote the initial weight of the guinea pig and Y its weight after the administration of the diet. The variable here is the ordered pair (X, Y), which is a two-dimensional numerical variable. The set of N ordered pairs, corresponding to the N guinea pigs in our laboratory, is the population.

In each of the above examples, the population consisted of a finite number of elements. One may also consider *infinite* populations, as in the following two examples:

Example 2.4. Let the maximum daily temperature for a certain town be the variable. Then the population consists of a maximum temperature for each day in the past, present and future, and is thus infinite.

Example 2.5. Let the variable be the weight of an aspirin pill (to the nearest hundredth of a gram) manufactured by a certain pharmaceutical company. Clearly, this population of weights also contains an unlimited number of elements.

Whatever the population may be, and whether it is finite or infinite, the investigator is usually ignorant about certain of its properties and thus prompted to make his observations. Ideally, the most complete information is obtained from observing the entire population, that is, from taking a *census* of the population. This is clearly impossible in the case of infinite populations and usually too cumbersome and costly even in those populations where a census is possible. It then becomes desirable to select a subset of the population which in some way can be considered as representative of the whole and to observe all the elements of this subset. Such a subset is referred to as a *sample*, and the set of observations obtained in a sample or a census is known as the *data*.

2.2. RANDOM AND NON-RANDOM SAMPLING

There are many ways in which a sample can be selected, the commonest of which will be enumerated below.

2.2 a. Simple Random Sampling

When each element in a finite population is given the same chance of being in the sample, the resulting sample is known as a simple random sample. If the elements are numbered serially, the selection is most reliably done with the use of a table of random digits, of which Table I in the Appendix is an example. A table of random digits is an array of digits generated in such a way that, for any given position in the array, the digit that occupies that position has an equal chance of being any of the ten digits $0, 1, \ldots, 9$, regardless of what digit appears in any of the other positions. As a result, a pair of adjacent digits is as likely to be one of the numbers $00, 01, \ldots, 99$ as any other; a sequence of three consecutive digits has the same chance of being any one of the numbers $000, 001, 002, \ldots, 999$; etc. To illustrate the use of such a table for random sampling, we suppose that our population consists of N elements and that the number N has three digits, so that each element in the population has a three-digit number corresponding to it. To select a simple random sample of n elements (n $<$ N) out of this population, we start at any point in Table I and read consecutive sequences of three digits until we have obtained exactly n different three-digit numbers none of which exceeds N, the population size. Then the population elements corresponding to the selected numbers constitute our sample. The same procedure can obviously be followed when N contains any number of digits.

Example 2.6. From a population of 6000 serially numbered elements (N = 6000), we take a simple random sample of five elements (n = 5) as follows: Arbitrarily choosing the digit in the 10th row and 15th column of digits in Table I as a starting point, and continuing along the same row in which it falls, we read the digits

      5 84643 42695 57102 38206 82957 82437 ....

The first four-digit number $\leqslant 6000$ in this sequence is 5846, the next is 4342; since the next number (6955) is larger than 6000, we delete the digit 6 and, for the same reason, delete the digit 9 following it, so that the next four-digit number not exceeding 6000 is 5571, then 0238, then 2068, making a total of n = 5 numbers. The population elements numbered: 5846, 4342, 5571, 238, 2068, constitute the sample.

2.2 b. Stratified Random Sampling

When a population consists of more than one category of elements and it is desired to have all categories represented in the sample in preassigned ratios, a simple random sample is taken from each of the categories (or *strata*, as they are called) separately. The combination of such simple random samples from different strata is known as a stratified random sample. Instead of taking a sample, for instance, from the set of all ages of patients at a London hospital, we may first wish to divide the population into the three strata: Londoners, British out-of-towners, and foreign, and then take a simple random sample from each stratum. This ensures, among other things, that the stratum with the fewest number of members is adequately represented.

2.2 c. Systematic Random Sampling

When a population is arranged or listed in some order that bears no relation to the nature of the characteristic observed, a systematic random sample is often the most convenient means of arriving at a representative sample. Essentially, a systematic sample is selected by first dividing the population into blocks of equal sizes, and then taking an element from the same position in each block.

Example 2.7. Suppose that we wish to select 50 names from the population of 3000 names of graduates of a nursing school for a study of careers in the profession, and assume that an alphabetical list of graduates is available. Since we are to choose 50 out of 3000, the sampling fraction is 50/3000, or 1/60; that is, our sample is to contain one name out of every 60 names in the population. We start by selecting a name at random from the first block of 60 names. This is done by choosing a number at random between 01 and 60, using Table I of the Appendix, as described in Section 2.2 a above. Suppose the number chosen was 17, then the 17th name in the next block of 60 (that is, the 77th name in the population list) is the second sample element, etc. Thus the sample will consist of population elements whose list numbers are:

$$17, 17 + 60, 17 + 2 (60), \ldots, 17 + 49 (60).$$

2.2 d. Cluster sampling

Some populations consist of groups or clusters of elements that are separated geographically or temporally and are otherwise similar, each containing a heterogeneous collection of elements. Rather than take a simple random sample of elements from the entire population, we can more efficiently select a number of clusters by simple random sampling from the set of clusters, and then observe all the elements within each selected cluster. To illustrate the method, let us consider the population of all the chest X-rays taken in a certain city. This population consists of clusters of chest X-rays taken at a number of different centers in the city, and a selection of a simple random sample of centers,   followed by the observation of all the chest X-rays in each selected center, enables us to reach a large number of observations quickly and efficiently.

Combinations of some of the above sampling techniques are also possible. For example Tomlinson *et al* (1973) describe sampling procedures in which they took systematic random samples of *clusters* of segments from the spinal cord, as well as systematic random samples of individual segments, for estimating the number of limb motor neurones in the human lumbosacral cord. An empirical comparison of the accuracy of the different procedures in their experiment showed no advantage in sampling individual segments over sampling clusters of segments, while the latter procedure has − of course − the advantage of efficiency.

2.2 e. Nonrandom sampling

Sometimes the investigator wishes to exercise his own judgment in the selection of a sample to be used for a particular purpose. In such a case, the interpretation of the sample observations must be carried out with caution, since a bias in the representation of the population may be consciously or unconsciously introduced in the selection.

Example 2.8. A case that may well illustrate purposive sampling is one of the early studies conducted by the United States National Institute of Health on the effects of tobacco smoking (Dorn, 1958). The investigators in this study found it convenient to limit their sample to policyholders of the U.S. Government Veterans Administration life insurance and among them to those whose policy was active at the end of 1953, since a follow-up of individuals in that group was considered fairly reliable. The sample was further restricted by non-response, and after the mailing of a second questionnaire to non-respondents, the investigators ended up with information on 85% of this special group. There was clearly no randomization in the selection of this sample. In fact, one can argue that holders of a Veterans Administration insurance policy on a certain date comprise a population and that the study was actually an attempt at taking a census and not a sample. On the other hand, since the purpose of the study was to investigate the effects of tobacco smoking on mortality rates, it seems reasonable to consider the observations as a non-random (or purposive) sample from a larger population of male adults in the United States.

Since health and medical data are frequently collected as part of a patient's record at a clinic, such observations cannot be considered as random samples. However, with a proper definition of the usually restricted populations from which these are samples, information derived from them can be used to maximum advantage in drawing conclusions about the corresponding populations.

2.3. ERRORS IN OBSERVATIONS

Whichever method of sampling is used, it must be recognized that sample observations are liable to various sources of error and that, as a result, they may not be as adequately informative about the population as the investigator may wish them to be. While some of the sources of error can be controlled, others, being inherent in the nature of the sampling process, are unavoidable, and therefore an understanding of the different types of error is necessary for a proper interpretation of sample data.

2.3 a. Sampling errors

These errors are discrepancies between characteristics of interest in a population and the corresponding characteristics in a sample drawn from that population. Consider, for instance, a population consisting of all potential responses by users to a new type of tranquilizer, and suppose that two-thirds of all users find the tranquilizer effective, while one-third find it ineffective. If a simple random sample is taken from this population, it is very likely that the sample will reflect the same dichotomy as the population, namely that approximately two-thirds of the sample responses will judge the drug effective. In this case, the *sampling error*, or the discrepancy between the sample and the population proportions, is small. But it is also possible for a sample to be drawn in which the sampling error is considerable, such as a sample consisting almost entirely of one category of responses to the virtual exclusion of the other. Although such an unrepresentative sample is very unlikely, there is no guarantee that it will not occur*, and if it does occur we normally have no means of judging it as unrepresentative because of our ignorance of the corresponding proportion in the population from which the sample is taken.

As can be seen from the above example, the amount of sampling error depends upon the particular composition of the selected sample, which in turn is determined by the chance mechanism of the sampling procedure. Thus the error can neither be avoided nor controlled and must be taken into account in using the sample data for the purpose of drawing conclusions about the population. Methods that deal with this transition from sample observations to decisions about the corresponding population, known as *statistical inference* methods, will be presented in Chapters 6 through 16 below.

2.3 b. Systematic errors

These are caused by such factors as faulty measuring or recording of observations, defective instruments, incorrectly calibrated instruments, or personal bias of the observer. No amount of statistical analysis can correct these hidden errors, and every effort must be made to avoid them both by adequate preparation before taking the observations and the exercising of care while taking them.

2.3 c. Rounding errors

This type of error arises in connection with measure data where the variable can assume values on a continuous scale, such as in the measurement of weight, length, pressure, etc. Barring systematic errors, the accuracy of observations of this type depends on the fineness of the measuring device and is usually reflected in the number of significant figures recorded in the data. If the degree of accuracy is so high that the data becomes too cumbersome to handle or the investigator considers it unnecessarily detailed for the purpose of his study, he can round the numbers by dropping a significant figure or more in each of his observations. Instead of recording a weight as 41.6 grams, for instance, he might record it as 42, thus introducing a rounding error of four-tenths of a gram. Fortunately, when a large number of rounded figures are combined in subsequent manipulation of the data, as in the calculation of their average, these rounding errors tend to cancel each other and are therefore not likely to affect decisions based on the data.

---

* Unless the sample is an unusually large fraction of the population.

2.4.   SAMPLE STATISTICS AND POPULATION PARAMETERS

A quantity calculated from the sample observations is known as a *statistic*. Several different statistics may be calculated from the same sample, depending on the type of information needed. If the sample is truly representative of the population from which it was drawn, these statistics provide us with good approximations to the corresponding quantities of interest in the population, which are referred to as *parameters*. It is our lack of knowledge about the values of population parameters that usually leads us to draw a sample and calculate the corresponding statistics. For example, the average age in a sample selected from the set of all ages of hospital patients is a statistic, while the average age of *all* the hospital patients is the corresponding parameter. Similarly, the proportion of Type O in a sample of blood types of factory workers is a statistic, while the proportion of Type O in the *entire* population of blood types at the factory is the corresponding parameter.

In order to interpret information provided by a statistic about the corresponding parameter, we shall be making use of what is known as the *sampling distribution of the statistic,* which is the probability law that describes the variation of the statistic from sample to sample in the same population. In Chapter 4, we introduce the basic tools of elementary probability and then describe some of the typical probability laws that will be used as sampling distributions of statistics in subsequent chapters.

REFERENCES

Dorn, H.F. (1958). The mortality of smokers and nonsmokers. Proceedings of the Social Statistics Section, American Statistical Association, Washington, D.C., 34-57.

Tomlinson, B.E., Irving, D., and Rebeiz, J.J. (1973). Total numbers of limb motor neurones in the human lumbosacral cord and an analysis of the accuracy of various sampling procedures. J.Neurol. Sci. *20*, 313-327.

CHAPTER 3
Presentation of Data

3.1. TYPES OF DATA

Raw data, or data in the form in which it is collected and recorded, rarely lends itself to ready interpretation, and in a census or a sample that contains a large number of observations the mass of raw data may even be more confusing than informative. To bring out the relevant information contained in the data he has collected, the investigator must organize it, condense it and present the summary in such a form that its essential features become evident. This chapter deals with the various methods that are commonly used in obtaining summaries of raw data and presenting them in the form of tables, diagrams and graphs. We shall see that some of these methods are more appropriate for certain types of data than for others, while methods that are generally applicable will differ to a certain extent in their application according to the nature of the variable, and hence of the data.

In one sense, all data can be classified into one of two broad classes: qualitative and quantitative. *Qualitative data*, also referred to as *categorical data*, consists of observations on qualities or attributes that fall into one of several categories. Thus observations on variables such as sex, blood type, marital status, profession, post-operative condition, degree of injury and extent of health education constitute qualitative, or categorical, data.

Quantitative, or *numerical*, *data* consist of observations on numerical variables such as: length, weight, pressure, temperature, density, count, rank, dosage level, etc. Numerical variables in turn are of two types, discrete and continuous. A *discrete* variable is one that can take only isolated values on a numerical scale, as in count data, while a *continuous* variable takes values in a continuum, as in measure data. In the latter case, practical limitations on the accuracy of measurement may force our observations to appear discrete, as when age is measured to the nearest year completed or height to the nearest centimeter. Nevertheless, data of this type is not discrete and must be handled by the methods appropriate to continuous variables.

While it is easy to distinguish between a qualitative and a quantitative variable, the classification is not always a rigid one, as some categorical data can be expressed numerically and numerical data can be placed in categories. If we are interested, for instance, in investigating the popularity of a certain kind of cough drop, we might inquire at a number of randomly selected drugstores whether, among the three leading brands, this particular one is the most popular, the least popular, or an in-between. Our sample would then consist of a set of qualitative responses which, if we prefer, can be expressed as the ranks

1, 2 and 3 on a popularity scale and treated as discrete quantitative data*. On the other hand, suppose we wish to find out how long a patient has to wait at an emergency room before he is attended to by a physician. The variable here is time, but for the purpose of our investigation we may be merely interested in whether the patient waits less than 10 minutes (short wait), 10 to 20 minutes (fairly long wait), over 20 minutes but no more than one hour (long wait), or more than an hour (very long). When a random sample of patients is interviewed, each is asked to state his waiting time in terms of the four categories, and the sample consists of a set of the statements: short, fairly long, long, and very long.

Data may also be classified according to the dimension of the observed variable, namely the number of characteristics that define a single observation. If only one characteristic is observed, be it qualitative or quantitative, the data is *univariate*. If two characteristics are involved in each observation, like the initial and final weights of guinea pigs in a feeding experiment, the data is *bivariate*. *Multivariate* data of 3 or more characteristics per observation can be defined similarly. A multivariate observation of the categorical type might contain, for instance, the following information on a hospital patient: sex (M or F), ward (surgery, medicine, etc.), hospital record (new or old), and diet (liquid, low salt, etc.). As can be expected, the organization and presentation of multivariate data becomes more complicated as the number of variables involved in each observation increases.

3.2. TABLES

3.2 a. Categorical Data

We first consider n observations on one variable.

Frequency Distributions. By far the simplest and most effective way of summarizing these observations is to list all the categories into which the variable falls, and then to count the number of times that the variable is observed in each category. This count is known as the *frequency* and the resulting table of categories and corresponding frequencies is known as a *frequency distribution table*.

Example 3.1. Suppose that the sex in a sample of 60 births taken from the records of a maternity hospital was observed as follows:

```
G B G B B B B G B G        B G G B G B B B B G        B B G G B G B G B B
G G B G B G G G G G        G B B G B B G G B G        G B B G B G B G B B
```

where B stands for "boy" and G for "girl". To condense the information, we first list the two categories of the variable (sex) as in Table 3.1 and then, taking the observations one by one, we place a tally mark against the appropriate category for each observation. (It is customary to draw the fifth tally across the four preceding it in order to facilitate the final count.) When all the observations have been entered, we count the tallies for each category and write the count in the frequency column. The column showing the tallies is now redundant and, although it is shown in Table 3.1 to illustrate the procedure, it is normally omitted.

*For more refined conversions, see, for instance, Abelson & Tukey (1959).

It should be noted that the total of the "Frequency" column provides a simple check on whether all the data have been classified, since this total must be equal to the number of observations in the sample. In other words, if there are k categories, and the frequency in the ith category is f_i, then $f_1 + f_2 + \ldots + f_k = n$.

Table 3.1. Frequency distribution of sex in 80 births at a hypothetical maternity hospital

i Category		Frequency f_i
1 Boy	𝟕𝐇𝐋 𝟕𝐇𝐋 𝟕𝐇𝐋 𝟕𝐇𝐋 𝟕𝐇𝐋 𝟕𝐇𝐋 /	31
2 Girl	𝟕𝐇𝐋 𝟕𝐇𝐋 𝟕𝐇𝐋 𝟕𝐇𝐋 𝟕𝐇𝐋 ////	29
	n =	60

Relative Frequencies. A frequency distribution can also be expressed in terms of the proportion of sample elements that belong to each category rather than in terms of their number. This proportion is known as the relative frequency, and we denote it for the ith category by r_i, so that $r_i = f_i/n$. Relative frequencies can often give a clearer picture of the distribution and are particularly useful when making comparisons among sets of observations on the same variable.

Example 3.2. In a study of blood component therapy at the American University Hospital in Beirut, Lebanon, Allam and Alami (1974) tabulated the number (frequency) of transfused units of each of several categories of blood transfusions in six consecutive years, beginning with 1968. For illustration, we reproduce their figures for the years 1970 and 1973 in Table 3.2. A comparison of the frequencies for the two years shows an increase in blood transfusions for all categories, but the change in the *pattern* of blood utilization is revealed only by a comparison of the relative frequencies, which show whole blood being used proportionately less, and blood components more, in 1973.

Table 3.2. Distribution of blood transfusions at A.U.H. in 1970 and 1973 by type of blood component

	1970		1973	
i Category	f_i	r_i	f_i	r_i
1 Whole blood	2850	76.37	4620	60.54
2 Packed Red Cells	448	12.00	1173	15.37
3 Fresh Frozen Plasma	99	2.65	259	3.39
4 Single Donor Plasma	119	3.19	698	9.15
5 Platelet Concentrate	38	1.02	360	4.72
6 Cryoprecipitate	173	4.64	434	5.69
7 Washed Cells	5	0.13	87	1.14
All categories	3732	100.00	7631	100.00

f_i = number of units transfused , r_i = relative frequency (percent)

Source : Allam and Alami (1974, Table 1).

Multivariate Frequency Tables. We can also construct frequency distribution tables to summarize multivariate data. Suppose, for instance, that we have observations on two variables one of which can be classified into r categories and the other into c categories. To summarize the data, we lay out a two-way table of r rows and c columns, each row representing a category for the first variable and each column a category for the second. Then we enter each observation as a tally into one of the rc cells according to the combination to which it belongs. This classification is continued until all observations have been entered. The tally count in the (i, j) th cell, denoted by f_{ij}, is then the frequency of observations that fall simultaneously into the categories represented by the i th row and the j th column.

Example 3.3. Using data from the United States 1970 National Health Survey, Westoff and Rindfuss (1974) report the responses of a sample of women to questions about the compositions of their families and their preferences as to the sex of the next child. We consider the responses to two of the questions as a set of bivariate observations and reconstruct the frequencies for their cross-classification in Table 3.3. One variable, the preferred sex for the next child, has two categories and these constitute the two rows of the table. The categories of the other variable, the predominant sex in past births, are represented in the three columns. Only the responses of women with at least one child are included in the table.

Table 3.3.   Preference for sex of next child and sex composition of past births in 4975 U.S. women

Past births

Sex preference		j = 1 all or most boys	j = 2 equal number of boys and girls	j = 3 all or most girls	
i = 1	boy	413	537	1484	2434
i = 2	girl	1671	513	357	2541
		2084	1050	1841	4975

Source : Westoff and Rindfuss (1974, Table 1). Copyright 1974 by the American Association for the Advancement of Science

In Table 3.3, in addition to the cross-classification frequencies, we have entered the sums of all the rows and columns. These sums, known as *marginal totals*, can easily be recognized as frequency distributions, the row totals being the frequencies of the row variable and the column totals the frequencies of the column variable.

In general, we use the notation: $f_{i.} = f_{i1} + \cdots + f_{ir}$, $f_{.j} = f_{1j} + \cdots + f_{cj}$, to denote the marginal totals.

Using these totals, we can obtain relative frequencies in three different ways depending on the type of information we wish to derive from the data:

(i) For each column separately, calculate the r ratios, $f_{ij}/f_{.j}$. These relative frequencies describe the distribution of the row variable in each column, and each column must add up to 1, or 100 per cent.

(ii) For each row separately, calculate the c ratios, $f_{ij}/f_{i.}$, which describes the distributions of the column variable for each row category. In this case, each of the rows adds up to 1.

(iii) Taking the table as a whole, we can calculate relative frequencies with respect to the total number of observations, that is, we calculate $r_{ij} = f_{ij}/n$ for every i and j. Clearly, $\Sigma\Sigma r_{ij} = 1$.

These three methods are illustrated in Table 3.4.

Table 3.4. Relative frequencies calculated from the frequencies in Table 3.3 (row and column categories as in Table 3.3)

(i) Relative frequencies of sex preference for next child (%)

Sex preference	Past births		
	1	2	3
1	19.8	51.1	80.6
2	80.2	48.9	19.4
	100.0	100.0	100.0

(ii) Relative frequencies of sex composition of past births (%)

Sex preference	Past births			
	1	2	3	
1	17.0	22.0	61.0	100.0
2	65.8	20.2	14.0	100.0

(iii) Relative frequencies of category combinations (%)

Sex preference	Past births			
	1	2	3	
1	8.3	10.8	29.8	
2	33.6	10.3	7.2	
				100.0

The above tabulation methods can easily be extended to the organization of data in more than two variables, as can be seen in the following example.

Example 3.4. Grizzle *et al* (1969) use a set of observations on 417 cases of surgery for duodenal ulcer to illustrate a general procedure for the analysis of categorical data. Three variables are included in each observation: the hospital in which the surgery was performed, the surgical procedure, and severity of the dumping syndrome. The authors' tabulation of the frequencies in a three-way table is reproduced in Table 3.5.

Table 3.5. Frequency distribution of 417 cases of duodenal ulcer operations

Hospital

Clinical evaluation of severity of dumping syndrome	1 Surgical procedure				2 Surgical procedure				3 Surgical procedure				4 Surgical procedure			
	A	B	C	D	A	B	C	D	A	B	C	D	A	B	C	D
None	23	23	20	24	18	18	13	9	8	12	11	7	12	15	14	13
Slight	7	10	13	10	6	6	13	15	6	4	6	7	9	3	8	6
Moderate	2	5	5	6	1	2	2	2	3	4	2	4	1	2	3	4
Total	32	38	38	40	25	26	28	26	17	20	19	18	22	20	25	23

Source : Grizzle, Starmer and Koch (1969, Table 5)

It is easy to see how relative frequencies can be calculated from such a table. For example, the total frequency for surgical procedure A is $32 + 25 + 17 + 22 = 96$. Of this total, $2 + 1 + 3 + 1 = 7$ cases, or 7.3 %, exhibited moderately severe dumping. At the same time, of the 105 operations performed at Hospital 2, 26, or 24.8 %, were of Type D, and so on.

3.2 b. Numerical Data

Frequency Distributions. Observations on a numerical variable x can be summarized in a frequency distribution table once a set of categories is defined for its values. Consider first a discrete variable, which takes the values $x_1, x_2, \ldots, x_k$. Listing these k different values of x (in ascending or descending order) as the categories of the table, we proceed as in the tabulation of categorical data by counting the frequencies of occurrence of each value cateogry.

Example 3.5. In an experiment on liver cell aggregation, Bikhazi (1978) has observed counts of liver cell aggregates in a certain suspension at different time intervals and different thresholds. His data for the 20-minute counts, rounded to the nearest thousand, were:

3	4	6	9	9	10	10	10	9	3	3	6	8	8	8	9
9	10	10	9	2	3	6	9	10	11	13	14	15	14	13	2
3	5	5	5	6	6	6	6	6	5	1	1	3	7	8	8
10	11	12	13	13	14	9									

For the purpose of illustration, we treat this data as discrete. We notice that there are 15 different values of the variable in the raw data, the smallest being $x_1 = 1$ and the largest $x_k = 15$. Taking these 15 values as our categories, we obtain Table 3.6.

Table 3.6. Frequency distribution of counts of
liver cell aggregations (15 categories)

Number of aggregates (thousands/0.5 ml)	Frequency
1	2
2	2
3	6
4	1
5	4
6	8
7	1
8	5
9	8
10	7
11	2
12	1
13	4
14	3
15	1

Source : Bikhazi (1978)

However, we may find it easier to interpret the data if the number of categories were smaller. This is easily done by combining more than one value of x in each category. Table 3.7 is a summary of the same data using 5 categories instead of 15, with each category containing 3 values of the count variable x. Comparing this table with Table 3.6, we see that, while the frequency column in the former is too detailed to exhibit any pattern, the latter shows at a glance that the frequencies gradually increase and then decrease as the number of aggregates reaches higher and higher levels.

Table 3.7. Frequency distribution of counts of
liver cell aggregations (5 categories)

Number of aggregates (thousands/0.5 ml)			Frequency
1,	2,	or 3	10
4,	5,	or 6	13
7,	8,	or 9	14
10,	11,	or 12	10
13,	14,	or 15	8
			55

Source : Bikhazi (1978)

In the interest of uniformity, when we combine values of a discrete variable into a category we must make sure that all categories have equal "sizes", that is, that they all contain the same number of values. Possible exceptions are the end categories which sometimes combine several values with low frequencies of occurrence. Table 3.8 is an example of a frequency distribution in which each category except the last contains only one value of x while the last category, being open-ended, contains an unspecified number of values.

Table 3.8. Frequency distribution of number of spontaneous abortions in 583 women participants in an international fertility research program

Number of abortions	Frequency
0	362
1	111
2	55
3	30
4	16
5	4
6	3
7 or more	2
	583

Source : Mroueh (1978)

We now consider continuous variables. If x is a numerical variable that takes values in an interval [a, b], we can construct a frequency distribution table for x by defining the categories as sub-intervals. Clearly, these sub-intervals must be so defined that:

their intersections are empty,
their union contains the interval [a, b],
they are of equal length (with the possible exception of end intervals), and
they are arranged in the table in increasing or decreasing order of x.

Accordingly, we shall use the half-open intervals of the form $[x_i, x_{i+1})$, $i = 1, \ldots, k$. with $x_1 = a$, $x_k + _1 = b$, and $x_i + _1 - x_i = w$, a constant, as the k categories. Subject to these restrictions, the choice of x_1 and w (and hence of k) are arbitrary. However, it is customary to choose a value for k somewhere between 5 and 20, depending on the sample size (smaller samples call for fewer categories), and to make $x_1, \ldots, x_{k+1}$ round figures whenever possible.

For a continuous variable, the categories for classification are also known as *class intervals*.

Example 3.6. The data below is length in centimeters of a batch of *Trigla hirundo* L. caught by commercial shore seine off the Lebanese coast in 1963.

11.8	10.8	10.1	7.6	6.1	10.0	10.5	11.6	15.0	11.4	10.2
8.1	6.5	10.2	11.2	14.2	11.3	10.1	5.2	10.1	11.5	13.4
10.5	7.1	10.2	12.1	10.8	7.6	10.2	14.0	10.2	8.4	12.0
9.7	10.3	11.5	6.6	12.0	9.6	8.5	10.9	12.8	5.4	10.7
10.8	4.4	15.5								

In this set of observations, the values of x range from 4.4 to 15.5. This range can be covered with 6 intervals, each 2 centimeters long, so we take $x_1 = 4.0$, $x_2 = 6.0$, etc., as in Table 3.9.

Notation. We shall use the notation n - m— to represent the half-open interval $n \leqslant x < m$ in which only the lower boundary is included.

Table 3.9. Frequency distribution of length in a catch of *Trigla hirundo* L.

i	Length (cm)	Frequency f_i	Cumulative frequency F_i	Relative frequency r_i (%)	Cumulative relative frequency R_i (%)
1	4.0 - 6.0⁻	3	3	6.4	6.4
2	6.0 - 8.0⁻	6	9	12.8	19.2
3	8.0 - 10.0⁻	5	14	10.6	29.8
4	10.0 - 12.0⁻	24	38	51.1	80.9
5	12.0 - 14.0⁻	5	43	10.6	91.5
6	14.0 - 16.0⁻	4	47	8.5	100.0
		47		100.0	

Source : Department of Biology, American University of Beirut

Relative and Cumulative Frequencies. As with categorical data, frequency distributions of numerical data can also be expressed in terms of relative frequencies, which are defined as $r_i = f_i/n$ for the ith category or class interval.

A method of presenting frequencies that is suitable only for numerical data is the method of *cumulative frequencies.* These are calculated for the ith category or class interval as the number of observations that are smaller in value than the upper limit of the interval. Or, calling the cumulative frequency for the ith interval F_i, $F_i = f_1 + \ldots + f_i$, $i = 1, \ldots, k$. *Cumulative relative frequencies,* as well as cumulative frequencies, may be obtained in this way. The calculation of all these frequencies is illustrated in Table 3.9.

Multivariate Data. The same cross-classification methods that were used in summarizing multivariate categorical data are equally applicable when one or more of the variables are of the numerical type. The only difference is in the definition of the categories. Table 3.10 illustrates this with data obtained from a catch of a species of crab off the Lebanese coast, with each observation classified by size and sex.

Table 3.10. Frequency distribution of size and sex in 993 specimens of *Portunas Marmoreus* Leach 1814

| Size (mm) | Sex | | Total |
	Male	Female	
5.0 - 9.0⁻	3	0	3
9.0 - 13.0⁻	5	0	5
13.0 - 17.0⁻	8	2	10
17.0 - 21.0⁻	37	16	53
21.0 - 25.0⁻	134	137	271
25.0 - 29.0⁻	203	220	423
29.0 - 33.0⁻	81	103	184
33.0 - 37.0⁻	18	12	30
37.0 - 41.0⁻	4	4	8
41.0 - 45.0⁻	5	1	6
	498	495	993

Source : Department of Biology , American University of Beirut.

Time Series. When observations or summaries of observations on a variable are recorded at successive points in time, the result is known as a time series. To illustrate the use of a time series in different applications, we cite a few examples from recent publications.

Example 3.7. The World Health Statistics Report contains records of the incidence of several infectious diseases in different countries. A given year is divided into months or four-week periods, and the item recorded for each period is the number of cases reported in it. The "point in time" for each period is taken as the midpoint of the time interval. The first two columns of Table 3.11 constitute a time series for the number of cases of measles in France over 13 four-week periods beginning with January 1976.

Table 3.11. Number of cases of measles reported in France in 1976

Period	Number of cases	4-period moving totals	4-period moving averages
January	210		
February	267		
		1100	275.00
March	350		
		1280	320.00
April	273		
		1390	347.50
May	390		
		1295	323.75
June	377		
		1146	286.50
—	255		
		795	198.75
July	124		
		439	109.75
August	39		
		216	54.00
September	21		
		194	48.50
October	32		
		309	77.25
November	102		
December	154		

Source : World Health Organization (1977, pp. 379-383)

Example 3.8. In a study of the effects of hypercorticoidism on the growth of juvenile mice, Silbermann and Maor (1979) recorded the weights of treated and non-treated mice at weekly intervals and calculated the difference (mean weight of treated mice - mean weight of untreated mice) which we reproduce in Table 3.12.

Table 3.12. Difference in mean weight of ICR mice treated with weekly doses of triamcinolone hexacetonide and controls

Age (weeks)	Weight difference (grams)
1	- 0.51
2	- 1.62
3	- 3.81
4	- 3.80
5	- 6.20
6	- 7.60
7	- 6.40
8	- 9.30

Source : Silbermann and Maor (1979, Table 1)

Example 3.9.   The time series shown in Table 3.13 is taken from a study by Efrati *et al* (1977) on the measurement of dry weight of blood lymphocytes in two classes of patients. Only the figures on morphology of the cells from chronic lymphocytic leukemia patients are reproduced in this table.

Table 3.13.   Cell morphology in patients with chronic lymphocytic leukemia

Hours	Morphology (mean % transformed cells)
0	1.3
24	6.6
48	9.03
72	23.67
96	30.78
120	35.13

Source :   Efrati *et al* (1977, Table 1)

It should be apparent from the above examples that, in addition to fluctuations from one observation to the next, the variable may exhibit a trend over several periods of time. The trend can often be made more apparent by a "smoothing out" of the short-term fluctuations as, for instance, by calculating a *moving average* for the variable. To define a moving average, we let x_i be the observation at time t_i, $i = 1, \ldots, n$, and suppose that t is measured in years. Then a three-year moving average of x corresponding to t_i is $(x_{i-1} + x_i + x_{i+1})/3$, $i = 2, \ldots, n-1$. A moving average can be defined for longer or shorter periods than 3, but it is always considered as corresponding to the midpoint of the time interval over which the average is taken. A 4-period moving average is shown in Table 3. 11.

Instead of a moving average, we may use a related quantity called the *moving total.* This is simply the sum of a number of adjacent values of x, considered as corresponding to the midpoint of the time interval over which the sum is taken. A 4-period moving total is also shown in Table 3.11.

3.2 c.   Mortality and Morbidity Tables

The mortality rate in a population is defined as the number of deaths in a year divided by the estimated number of individuals in the population half way through the year. If the population is restricted to a particular age group, the rate is known as an *age-specific death rate;* if the rate refers to a population with a wide range of ages, it is called a *crude death rate.* Mortality tables are tables giving death rates for a number of categories in the population. Thus we may have a table of crude death rates for several consecutive years, or a table of crude death rates for a number of different causes of death, or a table of age-specific death rates for a number of age categories, etc. Death rates can also be tabulated for combinations of categories belonging to several variables of classification.

Example 3.10. In a study of communicable diseases as public health problems, Cockburn and Assaad (1973) divided 32 countries for which the appropriate data was available into three groups according to their stages of development, and they tabulated mortality rates in each group for a number of different diseases. Table 3.14 reproduces some of their calculated rates.

Table 3.14 Mortality rates (per 100,000 population) for selected diseases in three groups of countries

Groups of countries

Disease	highly developed		less highly developed		developing	
	1957 - 8	1967 - 8	1957 - 8	1967 - 8	1957 - 8	1967 - 8
Respiratory infections	58.6	60.3	83.6	62.1	168.4	141.5
Respiratory tuberculosis	14.6	6.8	26.0	15.3	42.7	34.3
Dysentery	1.0	0.05	0.4	0.1	9.2	3.8
Typhoid fever	0.05	0.01	0.6	0.1	5.4	1.6
Diphtheria	0.3	0.01	1.2	0.1	2.2	1.0
Whooping cough	0.3	0.02	1.0	0.1	11.7	6.0
Measles	0.8	0.2	1.0	0.5	13.7	11.3

Source : Cockburn and Assaad (1973, Table 5)

Similar tables can be constructed to show rates of morbidity in a population. Although a number of different morbidity rates can be defined (see, for instance, Hill, 1971, chapter XIX, or Lancaster, 1974, chapter V), we mention only one example of such measures. For a given period of time, the number of illnesses that start during that period, divided by the number of persons in the population exposed to the risk, is called the *incidence rate*. If the size of the population at risk is unknown, it is estimated at a point half way through the period. Incidence rates, like mortality rates, can be crude or group-specific depending on whether the population comprises a wide range of groups or is restricted to a single one.

Example 3.11. Mantel and Stark (1968, Table 1) give a frequency distribution of discovered mongoloids born between 1950 and 1964 in the lower peninsula of Michigan,

U.S.A., classified by maternal age and by their order of birth in the family. Using the known number of live births for each combination of maternal age and birth order classification , they calculate cell-specific incidence rates as well as: crude rates ignoring maternal age, crude rates ignoring birth order, and a crude incidence rate   (89.5 per 100,000 live births) for the entire population of Michigan in the period 1950 to 1964. These rates are shown in Table 3.15. Adjustments to these rates, also calculated by Mantel and Stark, will not be taken up in this elementary discussion.

Table 3.15. Incidence rates of discovered mongolism by maternal age and birth order categories (per 100,000 live births)

Birth order

Maternal age	1	2	3	4	5 and over	Total
	(cell specific rates)					(crude rates)
Under 20	46.5	34.6	19.9	43.6	0	42.5
20 – 24	42.8	45.9	40.4	37.8	26.1	42.5
25 – 29	52.2	52.7	55.1	48.3	51.0	52.3
30 – 34	101.3	100.9	87.8	90.5	74.7	87.7
35 – 39	274.5	288.1	239.9	297.3	251.7	264.0
40 and over	819.1	725.6	866.1	976.2	857.8	864.4
Total (crude)	56.3	67.6	83.3	115.5	167.1	89.5

Source : Mantel and Stark (1968, Table 2)

3.3. DIAGRAMS

Graphical representation of raw data or of data summaries is an important aid to a better understanding of the data characteristics. Trends, symmetries, relationships, disparities and other features of the populations studied, are more effectively demonstrated in diagrams or graphs than in tables, be it in the early stages of statistical analysis or in final summaries and reports.

In this section, we describe a number of simple diagrams that are commonly used in representing frequency distributions of categorical data. As we shall see, these methods can also be used with numerical data when it is summarized in the form of a frequency distribution. Other graphical methods, applicable only to numerical data, will be given in Section 3.4.

The Bar Chart. This is a set of horizontal or vertical bars, each corresponding to one of the categories in the frequency distribution and proportional in length to the frequency of that category.

Example 3.12. The data in Table 3.16, concerning the distribution of health personnel in Poland in 1973 by profession, is taken from a report by the World Health Organization (1975) and presented graphically in Figure 3.1. In the figure, the categories have been rearranged in descending order of frequency. Although this rearrangement is not necessary, it gives a clearer picture of the relative sizes of the professional groups.

Table 3.16. Health professions in Poland in 1973

Profession	Number of personnel
Physicians	54,930
Medical Assistants	4,672
Dentists	15,091
Pharmacists	13,388
Veterinarians	6,600
Midwives	13,250
Nurses	98,593
Assistant nurses	19,051

Source : World Health Organization (1975)

FIG. 3.1. Bar chart of the data in Table 3.16 (frequency in thousands).

Multiple Bar Charts. When several sets of data are classified into the same categories, the frequencies for each category can be easily compared if they are represented by adjacent bars. However, since the total number of observations may be different in the different sets, we reduce all bars to the same scale by working in terms of relative frequencies.

Example 3.13. Tabbara *et al* (1974) observed the effects of an antibiotic (clindamycin) on infected rabbit eyes and compared the results with a set of controls using double bar charts. One of their charts is reproduced in Figure 3.2.

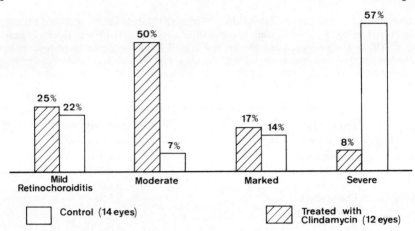

FIG. 3.2.   Histopathologic evaluation of retina in Example 3.13. Copyright 1974-75, American
Medical Association.

Composite Bar Charts.   Each of the bars in these charts is made up of components representing different subdivisions. To represent a bivariate frequency distribution graphically, we let the different bars stand for the different categories of one variable, and the
subdivisions for the different categories of the other variable, as in the next example.

Example 3.14.   The data of Allam and Alami (1974) to which we referred on page 13
is displayed by means of   composite   bars in Figure 3.3. To simplify the figure, we
have considered only three categories of blood transfusions:whole blood, packaged red
cells, and other.

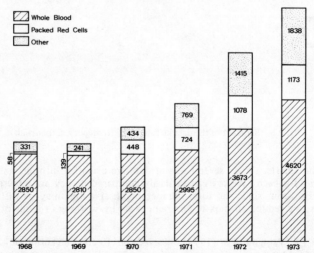

FIG. 3.3.   Number of transfused blood units at the American University of Beirut
(Allam *et al* 1974, Table 1).

The Pie Diagram and the 100 Percent Bar. These pictorial devices are particularly suitable for representing the proportions in the breakdown of data into k categories. In the first, the pie diagram, a circle is divided into k sectors such that the area of each sector (and hence its central angle) is proportional to the frequency in the corresponding category. The second is simply a horizontal or vertical bar which is divided in length into k portions proportional in area to the frequencies.

Example 3.15. Quoting *Vital Statistics of the United States,* Curnen (1978) lists five common causes of death in the United States in 1974 and their relative frequencies. Figure 3.4 shows a representation of this distribution in the form of a pie diagram. To illustrate the calculation of the central angle for each sector, consider the category "Diseases of the Heart" which, according to Curnen, was responsible for 38.2 percent of all the deaths. Since the central angle for the whole circle is 360°, the central angle for this category is (38.2)(360)/100 degrees.

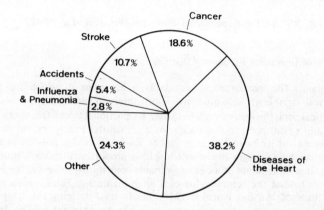

FIG. 3.4.   Causes of death in the United States in 1974 (Curnen, 1978, Table 1).

Example 3.16. According to the United Nations records for 1973, the world population (measured in millions) was distributed as in the 100 percent bar diagram of Figure 3.5.

3.4. GRAPHS

In this section, we describe several methods that are appropriate for the graphical representation of numerical data. For convenience, the methods will be grouped into 3 classes, depending on whether the data is in the form of: a univariate frequency distribution, a time series, or a table of bivariate numerical observations.

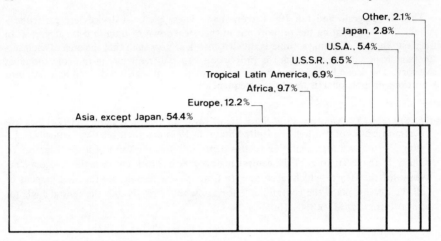

FIG. 3.5.   1973 world population distribution (Freedman *et al*, 1974).

3.4 a.   Graphs of Univariate Frequency Distributions

The Histogram. The histogram is essentially a bar chart in which the categories of the numerical variable are indicated on the horizontal axis and the frequencies are represented by vertical bars, the area of each bar being proportional to the frequency.

If the variable x is discrete and each value of it constitutes a category, the bar is drawn with the mid-point of its base at x, as in Figure 3.6 (a). It is also possible in such cases to replace the bar by a straight line whose height is proportional to the frequency, as in Figure 3.6(b). If several values of a discrete variable constitute a category, the bar has the mid-point of its base at the central value of x, as in Figure 3.7. Finally, for a continuous variable, the base of the bar coincides with the interval defining the category, as in Figure 3.8. In all of these cases, areas may be taken to represent relative frequencies instead of frequencies, if desired.

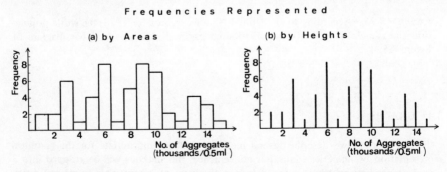

FIG. 3.6.   Histogram and line chart showing frequency distribution of counts of liver cell aggregates (Table 3.6).

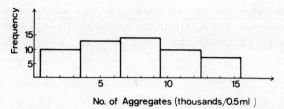

FIG. 3.7.   Histogram showing frequency distribution of counts of liver cell aggregates (Table 3.7).

The Frequency Polygon. A frequency polygon, which is appropriate for use mainly with continuous data, conveys much the same type of information as the histogram, though it may be a little more suitable for making comparisons. It can be constructed by connecting the mid-points of the upper sides of all adjacent bars in the histogram. To "close" the polygon, we connect the first and last points to points on the horizontal axis representing zero frequencies in the outlying categories. The frequency polygon thus connects consecutive points whose heights above the horizontal axis represent frequencies. The drawing of a frequency polygon is illustrated in Figure 3.8.

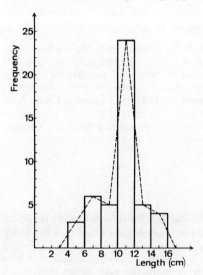

FIG. 3.8.   Histogram and frequency
polygon from data in Table 3.9, p. 19

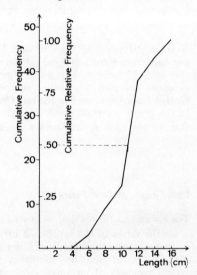

FIG. 3.9.   Ogive from data in Table 3.9.

The Ogive. The ogive, or cumulative frequency polygon, is also a line graph that is appropriate for use with continuous data. It connects consecutive points whose heights above the horizontal axis represent cumulative frequencies. Each of these points is plotted with the upper boundary of the class interval as abscissa and the cumulative frequency (or cumulative relative frequency) up to and including that interval as ordinate. Figure 3.9 shows an ogive constructed from the data of Table 3.9.

The ogive can be used for quick interpolation between plotted points. For instance, we can see from Figure 3.9 that approximately 50% of the catch *of Trigla Hirundo* L. were less than 10.8 centimeters in length.

Lorenz Curves. Suppose that the variable x takes values $x_1, \ldots, x_k$ with frequencies $f_1, \ldots, f_k$, respectively. Let R_i denote the cumulative relative frequency for the ith category expressed as a percentage, that is,

$$R_i = (100) \sum_{h=1}^{i} f_h/n,$$

and let S_i be the corresponding relative accumulation of the quantity x, that is

$$S_i = 100 \sum_{h=1}^{i} x_h f_h \bigg/ \sum_{h=1}^{k} x_h f_h .$$

If we plot S_i as the ordinate of a point whose abscissa is R_i, $i = 1, \ldots, k$, the resulting curve, known as a Lorenz curve, summarizes the concentration of the values of x by showing, at each point (R_i, S_i), that S_i per cent of the x values are concentrated in R_i per cent of the sample. Example 3.17 illustrates the construction and interpretation of a Lorenz curve.

Example 3.17. Taking the variable x as the number of male off-spring in a family, we use data from Reed and Reed tabulated by Rao *et al* (1973) in a frequency distribution of 2133 families. This distribution is shown in Table 3.17 together with the calculations necessary for finding the points (R_i, S_i) of the Lorenz curve. The curve, plotted from the entries in the last two columns of the table, is drawn in Figure 3.10. In this graph, a vertical line drawn at R = 50% meets the curve at S = 12%, which means that 50 per cent of the families account for only 12 per cent of the male offspring.

3.4 b. Graphs of Time Series

For graphing a time series, one uses the horizontal axis for time units and the vertical axis for the values of the variable. If the variable in a time series is a count (or frequency of occurrence), the resulting time series and its graph resemble a frequency distribution table and the corresponding frequency polygon. However, the variable may also be a measure, summary of measures, ratio, mortality or morbidity rate, or any other quantity.

Example 3.18. The number of still births in National Health Services hospitals in England and Wales from 1967 to 1977, quoted in the *British Medical Journal* (1978), are given in Table 3.18 and represented graphically in Figure 3.11. While both the table and the graph show a steady decline in the number of still births, the decline and its rate are more obviously demonstrated in the graph than in the table. Actually, the impact of the graph depends to a large extent on the choice of scale for the vertical axis. Although this choice is quite arbitrary, care must be taken that the scale neither exaggerates the trend nor masks the variations from one point in time to another.

Table 3.17. Calculations for Lorenz curve of data in Example 3.17

Class i	Number of boys x_i	Number of families f_i	$\sum\limits_{h=1}^{i} f_h$ c_i	$x_i f_i$	$\sum\limits_{h=1}^{i} x_h f_h$ C_i	$R_i = \dfrac{100c_i}{c_k}$	$S_i = \dfrac{100C_i}{C_k}$
1	0	590	590	0	0	27.7	0
2	1	615	1205	615	615	56.5	17.2
3	2	382	1587	764	1379	74.4	38.5
4	3	251	1838	753	2132	86.2	59.6
5	4	152	1990	608	2740	93.3	76.6
6	5	76	2066	380	3120	96.9	87.2
7	6	35	2101	210	3330	98.5	93.0
8	7	19	2120	133	3463	99.4	96.8
9	8	6	2126	48	3511	99.7	98.1
10	9	4	2130	36	3547	99.9	99.1
11	10	2	2132	20	3567	100.0	99.7
12	11	0	2132	0	3567	100.0	99.7
13	12	1	2133	12	3579	100.0	100.0

Source : Rao *et al* (1973)

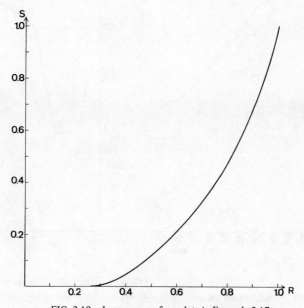

FIG. 3.10.   Lorenz curve from data in Example 3.17.

Table 3.18. Still births in NHS hospitals in England and Wales

Year	Number of still births
1967	11325
1968	10845
1969	9788
1970	9709
1971	9260
1972	8320
1973	7540
1974	6876
1975	6032
1976	5472
1977@	5209

@ Provisional

Source : British Medical Journal (1978)

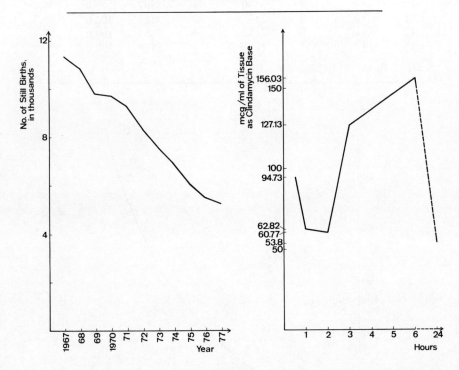

FIG. 3.11.   Graph of time series
in Example 3.18.

FIG. 3.12.   Graph of time series in Example 3.19.
Copyright 1974-75, American
Medical Association.

Example 3.19. In Figure 3.12 we reproduce a time series showing concentration of an antibiotic in the irises of experimental rabbits at certain post-injection intervals (Tabbara *et al*, 1975), each determination being the average from three animals. Note the break in the graph between 6 and 24 hours, which indicates the absence of any observations in this interval, while allowing the use of a reasonably wide scale for the available data.

Example 3.20. The monthly fluctuations in the incidence of influenza in two European countries in 1973 is compared in Figure 3.13 by means of the graphs of two time series. In each graph, the quantity represented on the vertical axis is the incidence in each month as a percentage of the year's total number of cases in that country. Thus the incidence figures are reduced to a common scale for comparisons and any significant difference between the countries in the *overall* incidence of influenza cannot be seen in such a graph.

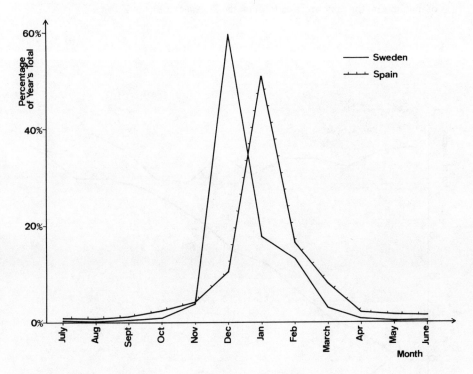

FIG. 3.13. Incidence of influenza in two European countries in 1973. Graph of time series in Example 3.20 (W.H.O., 1975, p. 100).

Z–Charts. A Z–chart is a plot of three line graphs derived from the same time series and drawn on the same pair of axes. One is the graph of the time series itself. The second represents, for each point in time, the cumulative total of the variable from the first point up to and including the one in question. The third graph is one of a moving total which, for each point in time, is the total of the variable over a specified number of periods centered at that point. The three graphs usually take the form of the three sections of the letter Z, particularly when the period of the moving total coincides with the entire period covered by the chart, as in Example 3.21.

Example 3.21. The number of deaths from motor vehicle accidents registered in Beirut, Lebanon, from July 1968 to June 1969, and the cumulative number of deaths, are shown in the second and third columns of Table 3.19. The column of moving annual totals was obtained from the records of the two-year period from January 1968 to December 1969; for each pair of consecutive months in the table, the moving annual total is the mortality count over a period of one year centered at the two months in question. For instance, the moving total corresponding to the point half-way between December 1968 and January 1969 is $11 + 5 + 4 + \ldots + 0 + 6 = 60$. The three columns of numbers in the table are used to draw the Z−chart in Figure 3.14.

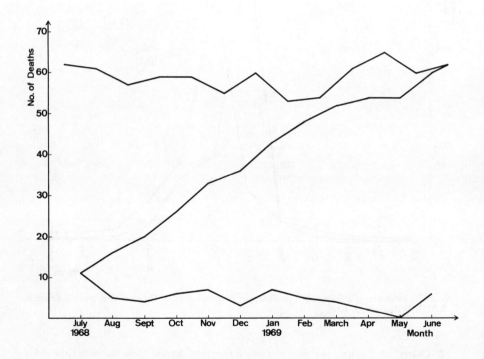

FIG. 3.14. Z-chart from data in Table 3.19.

Table 3.19. Registered deaths from motor vehicle accidents in Beirut, Lebanon

Month	Number of deaths	Cumulative number of deaths	Moving annual total of deaths
	(1)	(2)	(3)
			62
July 1968	11	11	
			61
August 1968	5	16	
			57
September 1968	4	20	
			59
October 1968	6	26	
			59
November 1968	7	33	
			55
December 1968	3	36	
			60
January 1969	7	43	
			53
February 1969	5	48	
			54
March 1969	4	52	
			61
April 1969	2	54	
			65
May 1969	0	54	
			60
June 1969	6	60	
			62

Source : Abou-Daoud (1970)

3.4 c. Graphs of Bivariate Data

The scatter Diagram. When pairs of observations on two numerical variables are plotted as points (x, y) on a Cartesian plane, the resulting graph is known as a scatter diagram.

The drawing of a scatter diagram is a useful initial step in the analysis of bivariate numerical data. If, for instance, the points fall on or close to a well-defined curve, a particular relationship between the variables is suggested by the shape of the curve. On the other hand, if the points are scattered with no apparent concentration, the diagram suggests the absence of association between the variables. Frequently, however, the situation is somewhere between those two extremes, and a certain amount of association is indicated.

Example 3.22. Table 3.20 summarizes the findings in a study of mercury concentration in fish caught off the Lebanese coast on May 8 and 13, 1977. The scatter diagram of this data (Figure 3.15) reveals that, in general, the larger fish had a higher concentration with roughly a constant rate of increase, thus suggesting that the relationship between concentration and weight is linear with positive slope. At the same time, the diagram shows a substantial amount of variation from this general rule, suggesting that factors other than weight of the fish have an effect on the mercury concentration. We shall return to this data for a fuller discussion in Chapter 14.

Table 3.20.´ Mercury concentration in *Mullus barbatus*
caught south of Beirut in May 1977.

Total weight (gm)	Total Hg (mg/kg weight)
57.6	.087
43.9	.047
75.1	.071
20.5	.031
29.5	.023
59.6	.087
30.9	.008
25.3	.031
43.0	.051
40.8	.016
40.7	.031
47.4	.039
26.3	.025
36.6	.031
28.1	.031
59.0	.087
44.5	.063
68.8	.055
55.5	.071
63.3	.063
56.5	.087

Source : Harakeh (1978)

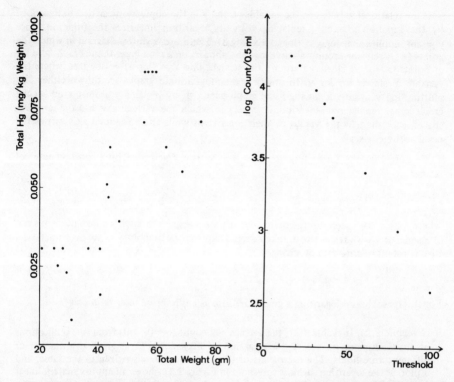

FIG. 3.15.   Scatter diagram from data
in Table 3.20.

FIG. 3.16.   Semi-logarithmic graph of data
in Example 3.23.

Linear Graphs. When the points of a scatter diagram suggest a linear relationship between the two variables, we can make a rough check on the plausibility of this type of relationship by holding a straight edge to the flow of points in the diagram. More refined
checks, such as finding the equation of the best fitting straight line and measuring the
strength of the relationship, will be taken up later in Chapter 14. Suppose now that the
rough check shows the trend in the diagram to be reasonably well described by a line
whose equation is $y = a + bx$. Then this indicates that in the population from which the
data was taken x and y are linearly related and that the rate of change of y with respect
to x is the constant b.

In some of the cases, when the points of a scatter diagram suggest a curvilinear, rather
than a linear, relationship, we can perform the same analysis if, by an appropriate change
of scale in x or in y or in both, we can make the points fall roughly along a straight line
on the graph. Two commonly used changes in scale that achieve this result, the semi-log
and the log-log scales, will now be described and illustrated.

Semi-Logarithmic Graphs. These are graphs in which one of the variables, say x, is
plotted on an arithmetic scale while the other, y, is replaced by its logarithm (usually to
the base 10).

If the relationship between the variables x and y in the population can best be described by the function $y = ab^x$, replacing y by its logarithm linearizes the function, since $y = ab^x$ implies that log y = (log a) +x (log b). Therefore, a scatter diagram in which the points (x , y) cluster around a curve $y = ab^x$ appears on a semi-logarithmic graph as a set of points (x, log y) clustered around the straight line Y = (log a) + (log b)x, where the variable Y stands for log y. In practice, semi-logarithmic graphs are drawn either by plotting log y against x on the usual graph paper, or by plotting y against x on special graph paper (called semi-logarithmic paper) in which the vertical axis has the numbers spaced according to the values of their logarithms while the horizontal axis carries the usual arithmetic scale.

We note that the linear function y = a + bx is characterized by a constant rate of change

$$\frac{dy}{dx} = b,$$

where dy / dx denotes the derivative of y with respect to x, or the instantaneous rate of change of y with respect to x. Likewise, the exponential function $y = ab^x$ is characterized by a constant *relative* rate of change,

$$\frac{dy}{dx} \ / \ y = \log b.$$

For this reason, semi-logarithmic graphs are sometimes referred to as *ratio charts*.

Example 3.23. In Table 3.21, the average cell count (per 0.5 ml) from five replications of an experiment on liver cell aggregation by Bikhazi (1978) is given at a number of different thresholds. The logarithms of these averages are also given in the table, and a plot of the logarithms against threshold in Figure 3.16 shows an approximately linear relation. The slope of a line drawn through the points in this semi-logarithmic graph would threfore measure the ratio between the rate of change in cell count (which is negative) and the count itself.

Table 3.21.   Liver cell counts in aggregation experiment

Threshold x	Count/0.5 ml y	log y
15	15028	4.18
20	12913	4.11
30	8862	3.95
35	7200	3.86
40	5756	3.76
60	2410	3.38
80	935	2.97
100	366	2.56

Source : Bikhazi (1978)

Log-Log Graphs. These are graphs in which both variables are plotted on logarithmic scales. When the relationship between x and y in the population can be described by the function $y = ax^b$, where a and b are constants, the relationship between their logarithms is described by log y = log a + b (log x), which is the equation of a straight line in the transformed variables. Consequently, if a sample scatter diagram plotted on a log-log scale shows a clustering about a straight line, this is an indication that the relationship between the two variables, x and y, is of the type $y = ax^b$.

This function too has an interesting characteristic. Differentiating both sides of the equation $y = ax^b$, and re-arranging differentials, we obtain

$$dy/y = b\, dx/x,$$

which implies that the model is appropriate for use with data in which the relative changes in x and in y are proportional. One situation in which this is true is the case where x and y represent two dimensions of the same organism and dx/x and dy/y represent their relative growth rates. In such applications, the equation $y = ax^b$ is called the *allometric equation* of growth, and b is known as the *constant of allometry* (Simpson, 1960). Example 3.24 is such a case, while Example 3.25 is an application of log-log graphs in non-growth data.

Example 3.24. Sweatman (1978) made a set of measurements on a sample of *H. dromedarii* female ticks randomly removed from their experimental hosts after a number of successive days of feeding. The lengths and widths of a sample of 26 ticks are plotted on a log-log scale in Figure 3.17. By inspection, the slope of the line, or the constant of allometry, appears to be approximately 5/3.

Example 3.25. In a study of particulate matter in some pharmaceutical preparations, Bikhazi *et al* (1977) and Shiatis (1975) examined several marketed preparations intended for intravenous administration and counted the number of particles that were found oversize at certain specified size thresholds. Table 3.22 gives the average of counts from five samples taken from a preparation they refer to as Product 1G. The data, plotted on a log-log scale in Figure 3.18, suggests that the equation $y = ax^b$ is an appropriate model for the relation between the two variables.

Table 3.22. Product 1G. Cumulative size distribution of
particulate matter in 0.9% sodium chloride solutions

Particle Diameter (um)	Number of particles oversize per milliliter
1.2	256
1.4	143
1.6	92
1.8	59
2.0	40
2.3	32
2.5	21

Source : Shiatis (1975, Table 3)

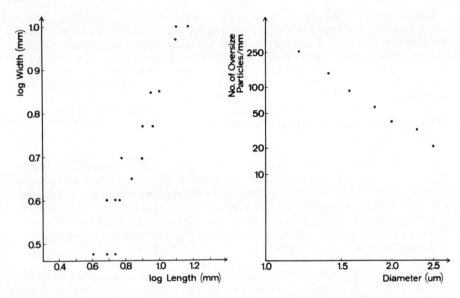

FIG. 3.17.   Log-log graph of data in Example 3.24.   FIG. 3.18.   Log-log graph of data in Example 3.25.

REFERENCES

Abelson, R.P. and Tukey, J.W. (1959). Efficient conversion of non-metric information into metric information. *Proceedings of the Social Statistics Section,* American Statistical Association, Washington, D.C., 226-230.

Abou-Daoud, K.T. (1970). Accident mortality in Beirut and suburbs. J. med. liban. *23*, 571-581.

Allam, C.K. and Alami, S.Y. (1974). Blood components therapy. J. med. liban *27*, 257-266.

Bikhazi A.B.(1978).*personal communication.* Department of Physiology, American University of Beirut, Beirut, Lebanon.

Bikhazi, A.B., Shiatis, J.A., and Haddad, A.F. (1977). Quantitative estimation of particulate matter in pharmaceutical preparations intended for intravenous administration. J. pharm. Scis. *66*, 181-185.

British Medical Journal (1978). Questions in the Commons. Br. med. J. 13 may 1978, 1287.

Cockburn, W.C. and Assaad, F. (1973). Some observations on the communicable diseases as public health problems. Bull. Wld Hlth Org. *49*, 1-12.

Curnen, M.G..McCrea (1978). Epidemiological outlook on cancer. Bull. N.Y. Acad. Med. *54*, 349-365.

Efrati, P.,Sokal, E., and Nir, E. (1977). Microinterferometric measurement of dry weight of blood lymphocytes in hematologically normal patients and in patients with chronic lymphocytic leukemia. Acta cytol *21*, 539-541.

Freedman,R. and Berelson, B. (1974). The human population. Scient. Am. *231*, 31-39.

Grizzle, J.E., Starmer, C.F., and Koch, G.G. (1969). Analysis of categorical data by linear models. Biometrics, journal of The Biometric Society, *25*, 489-504.

Harakeh, M.M. (1978). Mercury content of fish and seawater in Lebanon. *M.S. thesis*, Department of Biology, American University of Beirut, Beirut, Lebanon.

Hill, A.B. (1971). *Principles of Medical Statistics*, 9th ed., The Lancet Ltd., London.

Lancaster, H.O. (1974). *An Introduction to Medical Statistics*, Wiley, New York.

Mantel, N. and Stark, C.R. (1968). Computation of indirect-adjusted rates in the presence of confounding. Biometrics, journal of The Biometric Society, *24*, 997-1005.

Mroueh, A. (1978). *personal communication.* Department of Obstetrics & Gynecology, American University of Beirut, Beirut, Lebanon.

Rao, R., Mazumdar, S., Waller, J.H. and Li, C.C. (1973). Correlation between the numbers of two types of children in a family. Biometrics, journal of The Biometric Society, *29*, 271-279.

Shiatis, J.A. (1975). Quantitative estimate of particulate matter in pharmaceutical preparations intended for intravenous administration. *M.S. thesis*, School of Pharmacy, American University of Beirut, Beirut, Lebanon.

Silbermann, M. and Maor, G. (1979). Mandibular growth retardation in corticosteroid-treated juvenile mice. Anat. Rec. *194*, 355-368.

Simpson, G.G., Rao, A., and Lewontin, R.C. (1960). *Quantitative Zoology,* Rev. ed., Harcourt, Brace and World Inc., New York.

Sweatman, G.K. (1978). *personal communication.* Department of Tropical Health, American University of Beirut, Beirut, Lebanon.

Tabbara, K.F., Nozik, R.A., and O'Connor, G.R. (1974). Clindamycin effects on experimental toxaplasmosis in the rabbit. Archs Ophthal. *92*, 244-247.

Tabbara, K.F. and O'Connor, G.R. (1975). Ocular tissue absorption of clindamycin phosphate. Archs Ophthal. *93*, 1180-1185.

Westoff, C.F. and Rindfuss, R.R. (1974), Sex preselection in the United States: some implications. Science, N.Y. *184*, No. 4137, 633-636.

World Health Organization (1975). World Health Statistics Report *28*, 100-103 and 110.

World Health Organization (1977). World Health Statistics Report *30*, 379-383.

CHAPTER 4
Probability Distributions

4.1. PROBABILITY OF AN EVENT

Flipping a coin or throwing a pair of dice are familiar games of chance typified by an uncertainty concerning the observable outcome. In the case of the coin, the uncertainty is between its falling with one of its faces uppermost (Heads) or with the other face uppermost (Tails). If it is a perfectly symmetrical coin, physical considerations make these two outcomes equally likely; otherwise, one of them has a better chance of occurring than the other. In the case of each of the dice, there is uncertainty as to which one of its six faces will appear uppermost once the die has come to rest. Again, unless the die is a perfectly symmetrical cube, some faces will have a better chance of appearing uppermost than others.

Such uncertainties in the outcome of a trial are inherent in many of our less frivolous activities as well. They are encountered, in particular, at several stages of a scientific investigation, as in obtaining the results of a laboratory experiment or in collecting sample data in a survey. In fact, the process of taking an observation on a variable is not unlike that of performing a game of chance since the outcome remains uncertain until the observation is made. Consider, for example, the experiment in which a new drug is administered to a certain category of patients. For a particular patient, the outcome of the treatment may be one of several possibilities: there may be complete recovery, or only partial recovery, or no change in the patient's condition, or the drug may have an adverse effect on the patient. Each of these different outcomes has a certain chance of occurring, some a better chance than others.

A particular outcome or a particular set of outcomes of a trial is referred to as an *event*, and the quantity that measures the chance of its occurring is called the *probability* of that event. Thus, in the above example, we may speak of the chance of complete or partial recovery as "the probability of the event that the patient recovers." We write this briefly as P(the patient recovers) or, if the letter E is made to stand for the event "the patient recovers", as P(E).

Probability and Relative Frequency

Most people think of the probability of an event as the proportion of times they would expect the event to happen in many repetitions of the same trial. For instance, if told that the probability of recovery for a patient receiving a certain treatment is 75 percent, they would interpret this to mean that 75 out of the next 100 patients with the same condition and receiving the same treatment are expected to recover.

This view of probability as a proportion, if made more precise, can serve as a meaningful definition for the term. Consider a trial (like the flipping of a coin) being repeated many times under essentially identical conditions, and suppose that we calculate after each repetition the proportion of times that a certain event E (say Heads) has occurred *thus far in the sequence*. An important characteristic of this proportion, one that can be demonstrated empirically, is that after a large number of repetitions it begins to stabilize at a more or less constant value. In fact, it can be shown that the larger the number of repetitions, the less variation there is with each new determination of the proportion. If we now visualize the trials as continuing indefinitely, with the proportion of trials that result in E varying less and less from a fixed value, we take this fixed value as a measure of the chance that E occurs on any trial and call it the probability of E. In other words, *P(E) is the long-run relative frequency of the occurrence of E in indefinitely many repetitions of the trial.*

Although this definition of P(E) is a reasonable refinement of the layman's view of probability, it appears at first glance to be of little practical value. One difficulty is that it may be impossible to maintain identical conditions for the repetition of a trial; another, and the more obvious one, is that P(E) is defined in terms of an unending sequence of repetitions while one can make only a finite number of observations. If we assume for the moment that the trial is repeatable, then – in theory – the repetitions can go on indefinitely. The fact that we observe only a limited number of repetitions at the beginning of the sequence is not a serious shortcoming since, after a certain number of repetitions, the overall proportion hardly changes. As a matter of fact, we can use the relative frequency of E in a finite sequence of repetitions of a trial as an *approximation* to P(E); if the number of repetitions is large, we can be fairly certain that the approximation is good.

As far as the repeatability of a trial is concerned, what is important is that those aspects of the trial that are pertinent to the occurrence of the event remain constant throughout the repetitions. For example, if the trial consists of throwing a pair of dice and the event of interest is the outcome "double six", the manner in which the dice are thrown and the kind of surface on which they fall might be pertinent to the occurrence of a "double six", while the hour at which the trial is performed and the temperature of the room are not.

A more interesting illustration of repeated trials can be made in the context of random sampling, as in the following example.

Example 4.1. Suppose that we wish to investigate the smoking history of lung cancer patients in a certain community and that records for all the patients are available. We assume that the record of diagnosed cases contains, in particular, information about the number of years the patient was a smoker prior to diagnosis, and we denote this variable by the letter X. When a random sample is taken from this population, the sampling is equivalent to performing a sequence of repeated trials where each trial consists of looking up the record of one of the patients and observing the value of X. To insure that the trials are conducted "under essentially identical conditions", we must make the same set of values of X available as the set of possible outcomes for each of the trials in the sequence, and the sample must therefore be drawn *with replacement* – unless the population is so large that replacement is deemed to have no perceptible effect on the composition of the population.

Probability Calculations

From our definition of probability as a proportion, we can easily see that it must have the following numerical properties:

(i) For any event E, $0 \leqslant P(E) \leqslant 1$.

(ii) For an event E that is *sure to happen*, so that it happens in each repetition of the trial, $P(E) \doteq 1$. In throwing a die, for instance, one event that is sure to happen is that the face that shows up has less than 7 dots on it.

(iii) For an event E that *cannot happen* and therefore never happens in any repetition, $P(E) = 0$. Thus, if we agree that the only possible outcomes from the flip of a coin are the two faces, the event that the coin ends up standing on its edge has probability zero.

(iv) For any event E, the probability that it does *not* happen on a particular trial is $1 - P(E)$.

If we let C represent all the outcomes of a trial that do not belong to the event E, then C must occur when E does not, and the probability that C occurs is the probability that E does not. Therefore $P(C) = 1 - P(E)$. Such an event C is called the *complement* of E.

An event and its complement are one example of a pair of events that preclude each other in the result of a trial; if one occurs, the probability that the other also occurs is zero. Any two or more events having the property that the occurrence of one of them rules out the occurrence of any of the others are called *mutually exclusive* events.

The following three examples describe some events that are mutually exclusive but are not complements of each other:

(i) In the determination of a patient's blood group, the events "Group A" and "Group O" are mutually exclusive.

(ii) In measuring the weight of a newborn baby, the events "over 9 pounds" and "under 8 pounds" are mutually exclusive, while the events "under 9 pounds" and "under 8 pounds" are not.

(iii) When a medical student is choosing his future field of specialization, the events "Internal Medicine", "Neuropsychiatry" and "Dermatology" are all mutually exclusive.

We sometimes need to evaluate the probability that at least one of several specified events occurs. If the events are mutually exclusive, we can use a simple rule, called the Addition Rule, for calculating this probability.

> *The Addition Rule.* If A and B are two mutually exclusive events,
> $$P(A \text{ or } B) = P(A) + P(B).$$

A similar rule holds for more than two events. In general, the rule states that *the probability that one or another of a set of mutually exclusive events occurs is the sum of the probabilities of individual events.* Thus, if we are determining a patient's blood group, the probability that it is A or O is equal to the sum of the probabilities of A and of O. If we are throwing a single die, the probability that the outcome is an even number is the probability of "two" plus the probability of "four" plus the probability of "six".

The Addition Rule can also be used to derive a formula for determining the probabilities of events in trials whose outcomes are all equally likely. Take the throwing of the die, for instance. If the die is a perfect cube, all six faces have the same probability, which we denote by p, and all are mutually exclusive, therefore the probability that one or another of the faces appears is 6 times p. Since the appearance of one or another of the faces is a sure event, its probability is one, therefore $6p = 1$ and $p = 1/6$. Now consider any event in this trial, say the event that the outcome is even, and express its probability in terms of the component mutually exclusive outcomes. Then

$$P(\text{outcome is even}) = P(2 \text{ or } 4 \text{ or } 6) = P(2) + P(4) + P(6) = 3/6 = 0.5,$$

which coincides with what we would have guessed the probability to be if we were relying on intuition alone.

The above example illustrates the following general formula for calculating probabilities of events when all the outcomes of the trial are equally likely:

If there are exactly k outcomes for a trial and all k outcomes are equally likely, then for any event E,

$$P(E) = \frac{\text{the number of outcomes included in E}}{\text{the total number of equally likely outcomes}}.$$

As another illustration, consider taking a two-digit number from a table of random digits, and let B stand for the event that the chosen number is a multiple of 9. Since there are 100 equally likely outcomes (the numbers 00, 01, 02, . . . , 99), of which exactly 11 (namely the numbers 09, 18, 27, . . . , 99) are included in B, $P(B) = 11/100$.

In contrast to mutually exclusive events, where the occurrence of one reduces the probability of the other to zero, we now examine a concept, known as *independence*, where the occurrence of one event has no effect whatsoever on the probability that the other occurs; that is, for two events A and B that are independent, P(B) is the same number whether A occurs or not, and P(A) is the same number whether B occurs or not. This is illustrated in the following examples:

(i) In 2 successive flips of the same coin, the events "Heads on the first flip" and "Heads on the second flip" are independent, since the outcome of one flip does not depend on whether the other results in Heads or in Tails.

(ii) Let A be the event that the Johnsons' baby will be a boy and B the event that the Smiths' baby will be a boy. Unless one can argue that the sex of one of the babies is in some way influenced by the sex of the other, the events A and B must be considered independent.

(iii) In sampling with replacement from a population of colored and albino mice, events on successive trials are independent of each other, since the population being sampled remains the same from trial to trial. For example, the event that the first mouse observed is albino is independent of the event that the second observed is albino, and both are independent of the event that the third is colored, etc. In fact, since at each trial all the mice in the population are equally likely to be selected,

P(albino) = (number of albino mice in the population)/(number of mice in the population) regardless of what is observed on a previous or a subsequent trial.

(iv) If a card is drawn at random from a well-shuffled deck of 52 playing cards, the event that the card is a Spade is independent of the event that it is a Queen, since no matter what the denomination of the card may be, the probability of the event that it is a Spade is the proportion of Spades in the 52 equally likely outcomes, namely 13/52; likewise, no matter what suit the card belongs to, the probability that it is a Queen is the proportion of Queens in the 52 cards, or 4/52.

Given the probabilities of two independent events, we can easily obtain the probability of their simultaneous occurrence by applying the following rule.

The Multiplication Rule. If A and B are independent events,
$$P \text{ (A and B)} = P(A) \cdot P(B).$$

In the example of the card drawn at random from a well-shuffled deck of 52 playing cards, we have found P(Spades) = 13/52 and P(Queen) = 4/52. Since the two events are independent, we can conclude that the event of drawing a card which is at the same time a Spade and a Queen is (13/52).(4/52) = 1/52. That is, P(Queen of Spades) = 1/52. This checks with the probability of this event as calculated from the formula for equally likely outcomes.

The multiplication rule holds for more than two events also. In general, the rule states that *the probability of the simultaneous occurrence of a set of independent events is the product of the probabilities of the separate events.*

The following example, based on a simplified version of a population model, makes use of both the Addition and Multiplication Rules in calculating the probability of an event.

Example 4.2. Cook *et al* (1972) consider a dynamic model for a finite population of haploid individuals each of which can be classified as Type A or Type B, and where the type of each individual in a new generation is determined independently of all the other individuals and in accordance with the proportions in the previous generation; that is, P(any individual in new generation is of Type A) = the proportion of Type A individuals in the old generation.

Under the assumptions of this model, we now suppose that the present generation consists of 3 individuals, 2 of which are of Type A, and that the size of the population increases to 4 individuals in the next generation. Is it very likely that, out of the 4 offspring, there are 3 of Type A? To calculate the probability of this event, we proceed as follows:—

(i) We first observe that there are 4 different ways in which the 3 Type A individuals can appear among the 4 offspring. These 4 arrangements we represent symbolically as
$$\text{AAAB, \quad AABA, \quad ABAA, \quad BAAA,}$$
where the position of the letter in the sequence identifies the offspring having that type.

(ii) Since these four arrangements are mutually exclusive,
P(3 offspring are of Type A) = P(AAAB) + P(AABA) + P(ABAA) + P(BAAA), by the Addition Rule.

(iii) Since the types of different individuals in the new generation are independent, P(AAAB) = P(A) . P(A) . P(A) . P(B), by the Multiplication Rule.

(iv) From the proportions in the original population, we obtain P(A) = 2/3 and P(B) = 1/3, so that P(AAAB) = (2/3). (2/3). (2/3). (1/3) = 8/81. Similarly, we find that the other arrangements all have the same probability, namely 8/81.

(v) Finally, by virtue of (ii), P(3 offspring are of Type A) = (4) . (8/81) = 32/81.

The same procedure can be used to calculate probabilities of other events of the same kind, such as the event that 2 of the 4 offspring are of Type A, none of the offspring is of Type A, etc.

4.2. PROBABILITY DISTRIBUTION OF A VARIABLE

An event can often be conveniently described in terms of the value of a numerical variable. In Example 4.2, for instance, we may denote the number of Type A offspring in the new generation by X, and the event whose probability we calculated would then be the event that X = 3, while some other values of X would correspond to events specifying other compositions of the new generation. It is easy to see in this example that the whole range of possible compositions can be summarized in only five values of the variable — the numbers 0, 1, 2, 3 and 4 — which are listed with their respective probabilities in Table 4.1. In this table, as well as in the sequel, a value of the variable X is denoted by the lower case letter x. Since X can assume only one of these 5 values at a time, and since one or another of them is bound to occur, their probabilities must add up to 1. The way in which this total probability of 1 is distributed among the different possible values of X, as shown in Table 4.1, is called the *probability distribution* of the variable X.

Table 4.1. Probability distribution of the number of Type A offspring in a population of four individuals (Example 4.2)

x	P(X = x)
0	1/81
1	8/81
2	24/81
3	32/81
4	16/81
	1

In the above example, X was clearly a *discrete* variable capable of assuming only a set of isolated values on the numerical scale. Since it is in the nature of discrete variables that their values can be listed in some natural order, their probability distributions can always be represented in the form of tables like Table 4.1. As might be expected from the definition of probability as long-run relative frequency, a table of the probability distribution of a variable X should closely resemble that of the distribution of relative frequencies that might be constructed from a large set of observations on X. This expected resemblance between the distribution of probabilities and that of relative frequencies can be very useful as a check on the validity of a probability model when observations on the variable are available. Sometimes, the discrepancies between the two are so obvious that a visual comparison between the hypothetical and observed distributions is sufficient to discredit a model. When this is not the case, we can make use of a formal method for testing the "goodness of fit" of a hypothetical distribution to a set of data.This method will be introduced in Chapter 15.

The probability distribution of a discrete variable can also be represented graphically by marking the values of the variable on the horizontal axis and placing at each point a vertical line whose height is proportional to the probability of that value. Clearly, the sum of the heights of all the lines must be 1.

Example 4.3. In investigating the question of "clustering" in cases of childhood leukemia, Ederer *et al* (1964) considered a population consisting of space-time units each defined as a Connecticut town observed over a five-year period, and they recorded for every unit the number of cases that occurred in each of the five years. If cases did not come in clusters, the authors argued, the total number of cases in each unit would tend to scatter randomly over the five year period; on the other hand, the phenomenon of clustering would cause a large proportion of those cases to appear in the same year. So they took as their variable X the maximum number of cases appearing within a unit in one year when the total number of cases for that unit was a fixed number, say r. For different values of r, they calculated the probability distributions of the variable X under the hypothesis of no clustering and used them to make comparisons with frequencies obtained from the Connecticut State Department of Health records for the years 1945-59. One of the distributions obtained, the one corresponding to a total of r = 6 cases, is shown in Table 4.2 and again in Figure 4.1.

Table **4.2.** Probability distribution of X in the absence
of clustering (Example 4.3)

Value of X	Probability
1	.0000
2	.5184
3	.3968
4	.0768
5	.0077
6	.0003
	1.0000

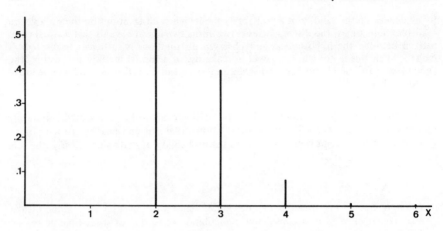

FIG. 4.1. Probability distribution of X in Example 4.3.

From the table and graph it is quite clear that, if no clustering is assumed, the most likely values of X are 2 and 3, and in that case we should not be surprised when observing a unit if we find no more than 3 cases reported in any single year. On the other hand, if we observe units with 5 or 6 cases in one year, we should tend to doubt the validity of the assumption that cases do not come in clusters, since under that assumption observations with such a large value of X have a probability of .0077 + .0003 = .008, or only 8 in a thousand.

When a probability distribution is completely specified, as was the case in Tables 4.1 and 4.2, one can calculate the probabilities of various events and use them in checking the validity of a model or in making predictions. Frequently, however, the probabilities depend on one or more unknown constants, or *parameters*, and in order to be able to interpret the probability distribution of the variable X the statistician must first obtain some information about the unknown parameters from a sample of observations on X. As an illustration of a distribution depending on an unknown parameter, consider the following simple hypothetical situation.

Example 4.4. Suppose that, for any given individual in some community, the probability of being colorblind is an unknown constant p, and that the incidence of colorblindness is independent for different individuals. Let A and B be two individuals in this community, and let X be the number of colorblind persons in this group of two. Then X is 0 if neither A nor B have this condition, 1 if A does but not B or B but not A, and 2 if they both do. It can be easily verified that the probabilities of these three different values of X are as given in Table 4.3. Since, whatever p may be, the sum of these probabilities is 1, Table 4.3 is a probability distribution.

Table 4.3. Probability distribution of the number of colorblinds in a group of two individuals (Example 4.4).

x	$P(X = x)$
0	$(1-p)^2$
1	$2p(1-p)$
2	p^2

When the variable X is *continuous*, its probability distribution has a different graphical representation from the one used for discrete variables. For a discrete variable, only isolated points on the line were possible values, but a continuous variable can — at least in theory — assume the value of any of the infinitely many points in an interval. An event is thus more appropriately described by an interval rather than by a single point on the line, and the probability of the event, instead of being represented by a vertical line concentrated at a particular point, is spread as a continuous area over the interval. This is shown in Figure 4.2 where the probability of the event A is the shaded area above the interval A, and where the total probability of 1 is spread above the entire set of possible values of X, which in this case is the set of all numbers between c and d. The curve whose height determines the area over any interval and hence the probability of that interval, is called a *probability density curve*.

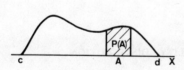

FIG. 4.2. Probability distribution of a continuous variable X.

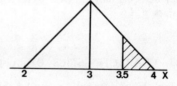

FIG. 4.3. Probability distribution of X in Example 4.5.

We again note the analogy between probability distributions and distributions of observed frequencies which, in the case of a continuous variable, are represented graphically by a histogram. If the sample is very large, the histogram can be drawn with a large number of very small class intervals, and the probability density curve can then be seen as the idealized form of a histogram constructed from an infinitely large sample.

The shape of the probability density curve for any particular variable depends on the probability model for that variable. This model is usually given in the form of a function y = f(x), called the *probability density function* of X* which, as in the discrete case, may depend on unknown parameters. The domain of the function is the set of all possible values of X, and its value corresponding to any x is the height of the probability density curve at that point. A number of different types of density functions, providing suitable probability models for a variety of situations, will be introduced in Section 4.4. We shall see that, in most cases, special tables will be needed to calculate areas under the density curve for the purpose of evaluating probabilities. This will not be necessary in the following example, where a very simple model is used just to illustrate the interpretation of a probability distribution in the continuous case.

Example 4.5. A hypothetical clinic opens its doors to patients from 2 to 3 p.m. every day and operates in such a way that a patient may be attended to at any time within an hour after his arrival. Let the variable X stand for the time at which a patient is served, which is the sum of his arrival and waiting times, so that the value of X is a number between 2 and 4. Now if we assume that the patient chooses his arrival time at random between 2 and 3 and that, regardless of when he arrives, the length of his wait is a random time between 0 and 1 hour, a reasonable probability distribution for X would be the one shown in Figure 4.3. The probability density "curve" in this case consists of two straight lines, so it is easy to check that the total area under the curve is 1. For this distribution, it is also easy to calculate probabilities of various events by using the properties of similar triangles. The probability that the patient is attended to after 3:30 p.m., for instance, or $P(X > 3.5)$, is the area of the triangle whose base is 1/2 and height also 1/2, and is therefore equal to 1/8.

It must be pointed out that, for a continuous variable, the probability of a unique value of X is zero. This is consistent with our interpretation of probabilities as areas, for the area above a single point is zero. Thus, in the previous example, $P(X > 3.5)$ is the same as $P(X \geqslant 3.5)$, and in general the probability of any interval is the same whether one or both of the end points of the interval are included. This is, of course, not true for a discrete variable. If X is discrete, $P(X > d)$ is in general less than $P(X \geqslant d)$; the two probabilities are equal only if $P(X = d)$ is zero, which is the case when d is not one of the possible values of X.

4.3. CHARACTERISTICS OF A PROBABILITY DISTRIBUTION

Probability distributions can be characterized by certain summary measures that are useful both as brief descriptions of the main features of a distribution as well as for making comparisons among different distributions. Some of the most commonly used measures will be defined in the following paragraphs.

4.3 a. Measures of Location

These are usually indicators of the central value or the "average" value of the variable in the distribution.

---

* It is common practice in mathematical statistics literature to denote a variable by an upper case letter and the values it takes by the corresponding lower case.

The Mean. Consider first a discrete variable X that takes k different values : $x_1, \ldots, x_k$. *The mean* value of X in this distribution, also called the *expected* value or the *expectation* of X, is defined as

$$x_1.P(X = x_1) + x_2.P(X = x_2) + \ldots + x_k.P(X = x_k),$$

which is a weighted sum of all the possible values of X with the weights being the corresponding probabilities. The mean is usually denoted by the Greek letter μ (mu), and the definition can be written briefly as

$$\mu = \Sigma \, x.P(X = x),$$

where Σ (sigma) is the upper case Greek letter that is used to indicate the summation of terms. In this case, each of the terms in the sum is the product of a value of X with its probability.

As an example, we calculate the mean value of X in Example 4.3, where X was the maximum number of cases of leukemia appearing in the same year within one space-time unit of 6 cases if no clustering is assumed. Applying the definition of μ to the probability distribution given in Table 4.2, page 49, we obtain

$$\mu = 0 + 2(.5184) + 3(.3968) + 4(.0768) + 5(.0077) + 6(.0003)$$
$$= 2.5747.$$

As can be seen from this result, the mean value of X is not necessarily one of the possible values that X can assume. Nevertheless, it can be taken as an indication of what value one might expect to find *on the average* in a run of future observations on X.

Although the above definition of μ does not explicitly utilize the familiar notion of the mean as an average, the quantity defined is in fact a population average. More precisely, if μ is the mean of the probability distribution of a variable X, then μ is also the arithmetical average of the population of all values of X, and hence is also known as the *population mean*. These two interpretations of μ are illustrated in the following simple example.

Example 4.6. Let X be a discrete variable with a population of 80 values, each of which is one of the numbers: 1, 2, 3 and 4, and suppose that the frequencies with which these numbers occur in the population are as given in the second column of Table 4.4.

Table 4.4. Calculation of the population mean

x	frequency	x.frequency	P(X=x)	x.P(X=x)
1	10	10	.125	.125
2	20	40	.250	.500
3	30	90	.375	1.125
4	20	80	.250	1.000
	80	220	1.000	2.750

To calculate the average value of X in the population, we first obtain the total as the sum of the third column in the table and then divide it by the number of elements. Thus the average is 220/80 = 2.75. Now imagine that we are to choose an element at random from this population and to observe its value. Since all 80 elements are equally likely to be chosen, the probability that the observed X is equal to any particular value x is the proportion of elements having that value x in the population, that is, the relative frequency of x. The probabilities are therefore obtained by dividing each frequency by 80, and are shown in the fourth column of Table 4.4. Finally, applying the definition of μ to the probability distribution, we have $\mu = \Sigma$ x.P(X = x) = 2.75, which is the same as the population average.

Clearly, the two calculations in the above example would have resulted in the same quantity no matter what the numerical values of X or their frequencies were, since the quantity calculated was a weighted sum of x values, and the weights — probabilities in one case and relative frequencies in the other — were identical.

The mean of a probability distribution has an important physical interpretation as well. In the graph of the distribution, if we think of the horizontal axis as a thin weightless rod on which the values of X are accurately marked, and imagine a set of weights placed at certain points on the rod with each weight proportional to the probability of that point, then the point at which the center of gravity of the system is located is the mean value of X.

So far, we have considered the means of discrete variables only. If X is continuous, its mean is also located at the center of gravity of the distribution, except that now the distribution is represented by an area. If a physical model of this area could be balanced at a point on the horizontal axis, this point would be the mean of the distribution. If the area is symmetrical about a vertical axis, the mean would simply be the value of X corresponding to the axis of symmetry. This is the case in Example 4.5 of the previous section; the probability distribution whose graph is given in Figure 4.3 is perfectly symmetrical about the line X = 3. Therefore the mean value of X, or the average of all the times at which patients are served at this clinic, is 3.

In general, calculating the mean value of a continuous variable is not easy. The definition of the mean of a discrete variable is here replaced by the analogous definition

$$\mu = \int x.f(x)\, dx$$

where f(x) is the probability density function of X, and the integration is over the entire set of possible values of X. But we shall not find it necessary to use this formula to evaluate μ, since f(x) is rarely completely specified; rather, we shall be mostly concerned with ways in which to use a set of sample observations to obtain information about μ. This is true in the discrete case as well. Our detailed calculations of μ for discrete variables with fully specified distributions were meant to contribute to a fuller understanding of the nature of the population mean rather than at developing skills in calculating it.

The Median.   Although the mean is by far the most important measure of location in a distribution, another commonly used measure is the *median*. The median is a central value of X in the sense that, if it were possible for us to arrange all the population values in ascending or descending order of magnitude, the median would fall exactly half-way along this arrangement. Therefore, in terms of the probability distribution, we might define the median as a number below which X falls with a probability of 1/2 and above which it falls also with a probability of 1/2. This is a meaningful definition if X is continuous, for in that case there is a unique point on the horizontal axis such that a vertical line drawn through it would divide the total area under the probability density curve into two halves.

If X is discrete, the concentration of probabilities at individual points makes it generally difficult to locate the median exactly. To cover this case as well as the continuous case, we define the median as a number m simultaneously satisfying the conditions that $P(X < m) \leq 1/2$ and $P(X \leq m) \geq 1/2$. For instance, in Figure 4.4(a), any number between 1 and 2 (inclusive) can be taken as the median m. In Figure 4.4(b), on the other hand, the median is unique and equal to 2 since $P(X < 2) = .4 < 1/2$ and $P(X \leq 2) = 0.8 > 1/2$.

Because its value is not affected by the magnitude of any individual x, the median is more appropriate than the mean as a measure of central location when the distribution contains exceptionally large or exceptionally small values.

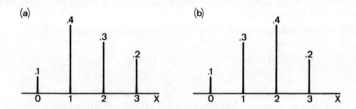

FIG. 4.4.   Two hypothetical discrete probability distributions.

Percentiles.   The mean and the median are measures of the average value of X. Other points of location that are sometimes measured are the *percentiles*. In general, the pth percentile of a continuous variable X is a value of the variable below which p% of the population values fall. In terms of the probability density curve, the area below the curve and to the left of the pth percentile is precisely p percent. Thus the median is the 50th percentile. In discrete distributions the percentiles can be found in a manner analogous to that of calculating the median.

4.3 b.   Measures of Dispersion

These are indicators of the spread of the values of X on either side of its average.

The Range.   The range is simply the numerical difference between the largest and smallest values of X in the population and is a rough indication of the extent to which population values may differ from each other. However, since the range is not affected by any of the intermediate values of X, little information about the probability distribution is provided by it.

The Interquartile Range.   This is defined in terms of two measures of location, the 25th percentile (known as the *lower quartile*) and the 75th percentile (known as the *upper quartile). The interquartile range* is the difference between the two quartiles, and it therefore measures the range of those values of X that constitute the middle 50% of the population. Because it ignores the upper quarter and the lower quarter of the population, the interquartile range, unlike the range, is not affected by extreme values of X at either end of the scale, and is therefore a better measure of the manner in which the more typical values of X are concentrated.

The Standard Deviation.   This is by far the most commonly used and most informative measure of dispersion. It is customarily denoted by the lower case Greek letter σ (sigma). For a discrete variable, the *standard deviation* σ is defined as the positive square root of

$$\sigma^2 = \Sigma\ (x - \mu)^2\ .P(X = x),$$

where μ is the mean of the distribution, and the sum is taken over all the possible values of X. The square of the standard deviation, σ^2, is called the *variance.* Thus the variance is a weighted average of the squares of the deviations of the X values from their mean, the weights being their probabilities.

In the case of a continuous variable, we have the analogous definition

$$\sigma^2 = \int\ (x - \mu)^2\ .f(x)\ dx,$$

where the integration is also taken over the entire set of possible values of X.

In Figure 4.5, we present two hypothetical discrete distributions for comparison. The variable X of Figure 4.5(a) has its mean and median equal to 3, and so does the variable Y of Figure 4.5(b), so that the two variables are equal on the average. On the other hand, we see that the probability that X differs from its mean by more than 1 unit is only .20, while the probability that Y differs from its mean by more than 1 unit is .60 — which implies that Y has a distribution with a bigger dispersion than X. This difference between the two distributions is reflected in two of the measures of dispersion described above, as can be seen in Table 4.5.

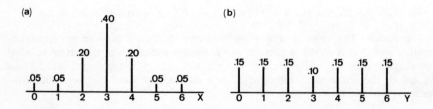

FIG. 4.5.   Two hypothetical discrete probability distributions.

Table 4.5. Three Measures of Dispersion for the Distributions of Figure 4.5

Variable	Range	Interquartile Range	Standard Deviation
X	6	2	1.30
Y	6	4	2.05

The Coefficient of Variation. When making comparisons among populations with widely differing scales of X a relative measure of dispersion is sometimes useful. Such a measure is the *coefficient of variation*, defined as

$$V = \sigma/\mu,$$

and which is clearly independent of the units in which X is measured.

4.4. SOME TYPICAL PROBABILITY DISTRIBUTIONS

In this section we define some types of probability distributions that are likely to be encountered by the investigator in the collection or analysis of his observations.

4.4 a. The Binomial Distribution

Consider a population of qualitative items, a proportion p of which belongs to a certain special category. When a random sample of size n is drawn with replacement from this population, the number of observations that belong to the special category is a variable, called a binomial variable, whose probabilities depend on two parameters, p and n.

Following are a few examples of a binomial variable, with the definition of the special category shown in italics in each case.

   (i) Suppose that the proportion of *male births* at a maternity hospital is 51%. Out of a random sample of 10 births, the number of males is a binomial variable with $p = .51$ and $n = 10$.

  (ii) In a batch of Vitamin C tablets, 1 per cent of the tablets have *weights outside the prescribed acceptable limits*. In a uniformity test, 100 tablets are to be chosen at random and weighed. Out of the 100, the number of tablets whose weights fall outside the limits is a binomial variable with $p = .01$ and $n = 100$.

 (iii) For a certain disease, the probability of recovery is 20%. In other words, 20% of the population of cases *ends in recovery*. Out of 50 patients chosen at random from this population, the number of recovering patients is a binomial variable with $p = .20$ and $n = 50$.

 (iv) In Example 4.4| above| (page 50), the number of *colorblinds* occurring in a sample of size 2 was a binomial variable with $n = 2$ and an unknown proportion p.

For any given pair of values of the parameters n and p, the probabilities of a binomial variable X can be calculated by the general formula

$$P(X = x) = \frac{n!}{x!(n-x)!} \, p^x \, (1-p)^{n-x} \qquad\qquad x = 0, 1, \ldots, n, \qquad (4.1)$$

where k!, called "k factorial", is defined as the product $k(k - 1). \ldots (3)(2)(1)$ for $k \geqslant 1$ and as 1 for $k = 0$. Program PROB1 of Chapter 18, which is based on this formula, may be used to obtain the desired probabilities. These probabilities have also been tabulated for various values of n and p (see, for instance, Burington and May, 1970). When n is large, binomial probabilities can be adequately approximated by areas under the "standard normal" probability curve, as will be described in Section 4.4 c below.

Since the probabilities of a binomial variable depend on the parameters n and p, so do the various characteristics of the distribution. In particular, the mean and standard deviation of the distribution are given by the formulas

$$\mu = np$$
$$\sigma = \sqrt{[np(1-p)]}.$$

Figure 4.6 shows graphs of three different binomial distributions with $n = 5$ and different values of p. The mean of each distribution is indicated by the symbol ▲. As expected, the smaller values of X are more likely when p is small and the larger values are more likely when p is large; when $p = .5$ the distribution is perfectly symmetrical.

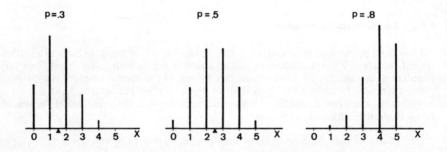

FIG. 4.6.   Three different binomial probability distributions with $n = 5$.

Of the two parameters of a binomial variable, n is usually a known number (the size of the sample) while p, being a characteristic of the population, is frequently unknown. When p is unknown, some indication about its size is provided by the observations in a representative sample. For example, a large observed value of X would suggest a correspondingly large population proportion, while a small X would suggest the opposite. Such inferences about p based on sample observations can be made more precise within the framework of the methods of statistical inference which will be described in Chapter 5. Inference methods relating to population proportions in particular will be taken up in Chapters 6 and 12.

4.4 b. The Poisson Distribution

Another type of distribution for a count variable X is the Poisson distribution in which the probability of any value of X is given by the formula

$$P(X = x) = \frac{e^{-\mu}\mu^x}{x!} \; , \qquad\qquad x = 0, 1, 2, \ldots , \qquad (4.2)$$

and where the parameter μ coincides with the mean value of X. In this model, the variable X is the number of occurrences of a rare event over a specified unit of time or space. The event is "rare" in the sense that, if the unit is divided into a very large number n of small components, the probability p that the event occurs in any one such component is exceedingly small. The distribution is therefore like that of a binomial variable with large n, small p, and mean value $\mu = np$. In fact, it can be shown that if we replace p in the binomial probability formula (4.1) by μ/n and take the limit of that probability as n $\rightarrow\infty$, the result is the Poisson probability (4.2).

Following are some examples of chance phenomena in which the Poisson model has been found appropriate:

(i)   The number of clusters of organisms appearing on the surface of a slide culture (see, for example, Thomas *et al*, 1972).
(ii) The number of petroleum reservoirs occurring in a geographical region (see, for example, Uhler *et al*, 1970).
(iii) The number of patients admitted or discharged in a large hospital (see, for example, Duncan and Curnow, 1978).
(iv) The number of counts of α–particles falling on a detector from a steady source (see, for example, Parratt, 1961, p. 215).
(v)   The number of occurrences of a certain symptom in a patient during a specified interval of time (see, for example, Layard and Arvesen, 1978).

One characteristic of a Poisson variable is that its mean and variance are both equal to the parameter of the distribution. In other words,

$$\sigma^2 = \mu \; .$$

If μ is known, the Poisson probability can be calculated by means of formula (4.2). Tables are also available giving probabilities corresponding to various values of μ (see, for instance, Pearson and Hartley, 1966, Table 39). When μ is not known and some information about it is sought, the standard methods of statistical inference given in Chapter 8 can be employed if a large sample of observations on X is available.

Figure 4.7 shows graphs of three different Poisson distributions. We note that the distribution with the largest μ in the figure has the largest amount of dispersion, which is consistent with the fact that $\sigma^2 = \mu$.

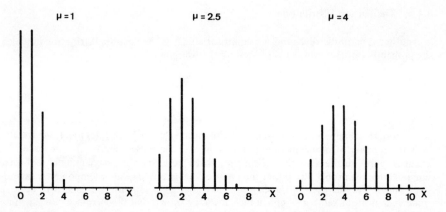

FIG. 4.7. Three different Poisson probability distributions.

4.4 c. The Normal Distribution

Also known as the Gaussian distribution, this is the most widely used probability distribution in statistics. Unlike the two variables introduced in earlier paragraphs, the normal
variable is continuous, and its probabilities are represented graphically by areas under a
probability density curve. For a normal variable with mean μ and standard deviation σ,
the probability density function has the form

$$f(x) = \frac{1}{\sigma\sqrt{2\pi}}\ e^{-\frac{1}{2}(x-\mu)^2/\sigma^2} \tag{4.3}$$

so that μ and σ are the parameters of the distribution. In Figure 4.8(a), we display a number of different normal density curves with different combinations of parameter values.
The distribution whose mean is zero and standard deviation is one is known as the *standard normal.*

The normal distribution has proved to be an appropriate model for a very large number
of different kinds of variables, particularly when the observations on those variables are
of the measurement type. Its use, however, goes far beyond providing probability models
for sets of observations, as will become evident in later chapters.

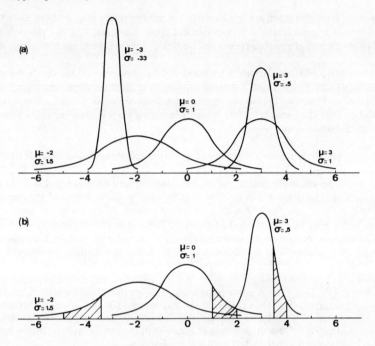

FIG. 4.8. Normal density curves.

The following examples illustrate the versatility of the normal distribution by citing some of its common uses.

(i) Heights of individuals in a population, their weights, and several other measurable biological characteristics, are usually well described by the normal distribution.

(ii) The I.Q.'s in a cross-sectional population, the scores on a standardized test, and other quantifications of abilities or achievements have also been found to conform to the normal model.

(iii) Random errors in measurements, which are either positive or negative deviations from the true quantity measured, can be taken as normally distributed about a zero mean. In fact, the normal density curve has also been known as the "error curve" and areas under the standard normal curve as the "error function".

(iv) The normal distribution also provides a reasonably good approximation to probabilities of discrete variables when certain conditions are satisfied, as will be specified in later paragraphs.

(v) The arithmetical average of a large set of observations on a variable is approximately normally distributed. This fact is true for most of the known populations, continuous or discrete, and will be utilized in Chapter 8.

Some properties of the normal distribution can be deduced from Equation (4.3) and from the graphs in Figure 4.8. It is obvious, for example, that the distribution is symmetrical with respect to the mean, that the mean and median coincide, and that values of X that are far from the mean are less likely to occur than values near it. Also, since the density curve for any particular X is symmetrical about the mean, any two intervals that are equal in length and at equal distances on opposite sides of the mean have equal probabilities.

One property of the distribution that may not be so obvious is that the probabilities of the different sets of values of X depend only on how far those values are from μ in terms of σ. Thus, in Figure 4.8(b), *all the three shaded areas are equal*, since each represents the probability that the variable differs from its mean by no less than one and no more than two standard deviations.

When a variable is referred to its mean as origin and measured in units of its standard deviation, we call it "standardized". In view of the property of normal distributions stated in the previous paragraph, the probabilities for any normal variable X with mean μ and standard deviation σ can be expressed in terms of probabilities of the *standardized* variable $Z = (X - \mu)/\sigma$. Now Z has the standard normal distribution, and areas under its density curve have been extensively tabulated. Table II in the Appendix, which is a partial reproduction of more extensive tables, gives areas under the standard normal curve to the right of a sequence of positive values of Z. Its use in calculating probabilities for a non-standard normal variable is illustrated in the following example.

Example 4.7. In a certain adult population, the immunoglobulin level X, measured as the concentration of IgG in mg/1000 ml, has mean 1100 and standard deviation 350. Assuming that X is normally distributed in the population, we can calculate the probability (indicated by the shaded area in Figure 4.9) that an individual chosen at random from this population has an IgG level less than 500 as

$$P(X < 500) = P \left(\frac{X - 1100}{350} < \frac{500 - 1100}{350} \right)$$

$= P(Z < -1.71)$
$= P(Z > 1.71)$ because of symmetry
$= .0436$, or 4.36%.

4.36% can also be interpreted as the proportion of individuals in the population whose IgG level X is below 500 mg/1000 ml.

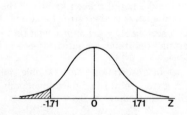

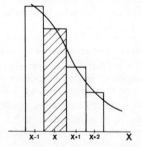

FIG. 4.9.   Area corresponding to   FIG. 4.10.   Approximating P(X = x) by
P(X < 500) in Example 4.7.   area under a normal curve.

As can be verified from Table II, more than two-thirds of a normal population fall within one standard deviation of the mean. In fact, $P(-1 < Z < 1) = .6826$. Moreover, $P(-2 < Z < 2) =. 9544$ and $P(-3 < Z < 3) =. 9974$, the latter implying that only a very small fraction of the population (26 in 10,000) differs from its mean by 3 standard deviations or more. For numbers larger than 3, the "tail probabilities", which are the probabilities of numerically larger values of Z, are even smaller than this fraction.

The Normal Approximation to the Binomial The areas under the standard normal curve can be used to approximate probabilities of a binomial variable, and the approximation is particularly good when n is large. The approximation can perhaps be better understood if we first modify the graphical representation of the binomial distribution, replacing each probability line which is concentrated at a point x by a vertical bar of the same height and with base extending from $x - 1/2$ to $x + 1/2$. Since the height of the bar is equal to $P(X = x)$, so is its area. When this is done for all x, the graph becomes a histogram whose total area is one. If a normal curve with mean np and variance $np(1-p)$ is drawn over the histogram, its area is also one, and the areas of portions of the histogram can be approximated by the corresponding areas under the curve, as in Figure 4.10. For example, $P(X = x)$ is approximately the area under the normal curve between $X = x-1/2$ and $X = x + 1/2$; similarly, $P(X > x)$ is approximately the area to the right of the line $X = x + 1/2$ under the normal curve. This addition or subtraction of half a unit is called the "correction for continuity". Once this correction has been made, the variable is standardized and Table II is used in calculating the probability, as in the next example.

Example 4.8. Let Y be a binomial variable with $n = 20$ and $p = .6$, so that $\mu = 12$ and $\sigma = 2.19$. To approximate the probability $P(10 \leqslant Y \leqslant 15)$, we apply the correction for continuity to include, in this case, both end points of the interval, and calculate the area under the curve and over the interval: $9.5 \leqslant Y \leqslant 15.5$. Now $P(9.5 \leqslant Y \leqslant 15.5)$ is approximately equal to.

$$P(\frac{9.5-12}{2.19} \leqslant Z \leqslant \frac{15.5-12}{2.19}),$$

where Z is standard normal. This is $P(-1.14 \leqslant Z \leqslant 1.60) = 1-(.0548 + .1271) = .8181$.

The exact probability of this event, on the other hand, can be obtained from tables of the binomial distribution, or by using Program PROB2 of Chapter 18, and is found to be .8194, which differs very little from the approximated value. The normal approximation to binomial probabilities can also be obtained by an application of Program PROB3, as described and illustrated in Chapter 18.

In the above example, the normal approximation yielded a probability that was accurate to two decimal places, and one might ask whether the approximation is always as good as this. One rule of thumb that is useful in this case is to *approximate the binomial probabilities by the normal distribution if the smaller of the quantities np and n(1 – p) is at least 5.* In the above example, the smaller product was 8.

The Normal Approximation to the Poisson. Poisson probabilities can also be approximated by areas under the normal curve in a manner analogous to the approximation of binomial probabilites. To approximate, for instance, the probability that a Poisson variable with parameter $\mu = 9$ (and hence $\sigma = 3$) is below 10, we write

$$P(X < 10) \cong P(Z < \frac{9.5 - 9}{3}) = P(Z < .17) = 1 - .4325 = .5675.$$

The exact probability obtained from Poisson probability tables is .5874 which shows the approximation to be in error by about 4%. Better approximations can be obtained when the Poisson parameter is larger than its value in this example and, in general, the larger the parameter is, the better the approximation — as might be guessed from the increased tendency towards symmetry with increased μ in Figure 4.7. The normal approximation to Poisson probabilities can also be obtained by an application of Program PROB4, as described and illustrated in Chapter 18.

4.4 d. The Exponential Dsitribution

This distribution is also of the continuous type, but the variable is such that negative values are not possible. Its probability density function is given by the equation

$$f(x) = \frac{1}{\mu} e^{-x/\mu}, \qquad\qquad x \geqslant 0. \qquad\qquad (4.4)$$

It can be easily shown that both the mean and the standard deviation of X are equal to the parameter μ. In Figure 4.11 we present some exponential probability density curves corresponding to different values of the parameter.

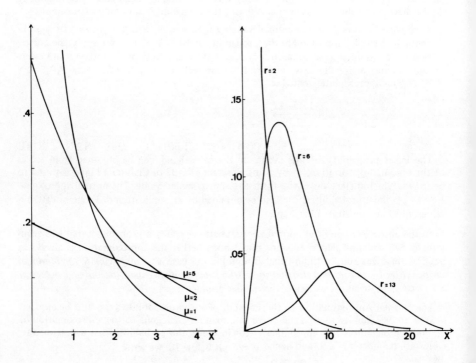

FIG. 4.11. Exponential density curves.   FIG. 4.12. Chi-square density curves.

Some examples of variables for which the exponential model has been found appropriate are the following:

(i) X as survival time, e.g. the time from the initiation of a specific treatment, or from diagnosis, to death. The parameter may differ from disease to disease or from patient to patient (see, for example, Feigl and Zelen, 1965).

(ii) X as a physical quantity, e.g. the volume of fluid between consecutive blood cells of a certain type passing through the aperture in a Coulter counter (see, for example, Mazumdar and Kussmaul, 1967).

(iii) X as time elapsed before start of deterioration in material due to fungal attack (see, for example, Maritz, 1957).

No tables are needed for calculating probabilities of this variable. By straightforward integration it is easy to see that, for any given x, $P(X > x) = e^{-x/\mu}$. If μ is unknown and a sample of observations on X is available, an approximation for this probability can be obtained if the parameter is replaced by an estimate derived from the sample (for estimating a mean, see Chapter 8).

The four distributions described in the previous paragraphs, while not exhaustive, cover a wide variety of types of observations. Some, particularly the normal, are also useful as *sampling distributions*, which are probability distributions of variable quantities that can be calculated from the set of observations, rather than directly observed. Such quantities are called *statistics*. The following three distributions are mainly of interest as sampling distributions of statistics and will be frequently referred to in future chapters.

4.4. e. The Chi-Square Distribution

The sum of squares of r independent standard normal variables is a variable whose probability distribution is known as Chi-square and denoted simply by the symbol χ^2. Its probability density function, which we find no need to reproduce here, depends on only one parameter, r, called its *degrees of freedom**.

By its definition, the Chi-square variable can take only non-negative values. Also, it can be shown that, if Y is a Chi-square variable with r degrees of freedom, $E(Y) = r$ and $\sigma(Y) = \sqrt{2r}$.

Examples of some Chi-square density curves are shown in Figure 4.12 for different values of r, the degrees of freedom (which we briefly denote by d.f.). When $r = 2$, the distribution coincides with that of the exponential variable with mean 2. As suggested by these graphs, the distribution becomes more nearly symmetrical as r increases.

Table III in the Appendix can be used to find some of the percentiles of χ^2 variables with r anywhere from 1 to 30 as well as for some selected larger values of r. For each value of r (each row of the table), and each specified probability P (each column of the table), we can read *the value of χ^2 that is exceeded with probability P*. For example, corresponding to the row $r = 12$ and the column $P = .25$, we find a χ^2 value of

---

* The notion of "degrees of freedom" will be enlarged upon in Chapter 7, Section 7.2.

14.845. This means that if Y is a Chi-square variable with 12 degrees of freedom, $P(Y > 14.845) = .25$ or that 14.845 is the 75th percentile (or upper quartile) of this particular Chi-square distribution.

For degrees of freedom larger than those tabulated, we can use a normal approximation to the Chi-square distribution, since it is known that, for a χ^2 variable Y with large r, $X = \sqrt{(2Y)} - \sqrt{(2r-1)}$ is approximately standard normal (see, for instance, Kendall and Stuart, 1969, p. 371).

Example 4.9. Suppose that we want to find the value y of a χ^2 variable Y with 75 degrees of freedom such that $P(Y > y) = .25$ Using the approximation of the previous paragraph, we rewrite the condition as

$$0.25 = P(\sqrt{(2Y)} > \sqrt{(2y)})$$
$$= P(\sqrt{(2Y)} - \sqrt{149} > \sqrt{(2y)} - \sqrt{149})$$
$$\cong P(Z > \sqrt{(2y)} - 12.2066)$$

where Z is the standard normal variable. From the normal tables (Table II in the Appendix), we find that $\sqrt{(2y)} - 12.2066 = .6745$, and therefore $y = (12.8811)^2/2 = 82.96$. By comparison, interpolation between $r = 70$ and $r = 80$ in Table III yields $y = 82.86$.

4.4 f. The t distribution

This variable, usually referred to as "Student's t", is also related to the standard normal variable. In fact, if X is standard normal, and Y is an independently distributed χ^2 variable with r d.f., then

$$T = \frac{X}{\sqrt{Y/r}}$$

has Student's t-distribution with r degrees of freedom. It follows that the t-distribution has only one parameter, namely its degrees of freedom, r.

Some properties of this distribution are: (i) It is symmetrical about zero, which is its mean. (ii) Its variance is equal to $r/(r-2)$. (iii) The probability density curve is very similar to that of the standard normal curve, as can be seen in Figure 4.13, where, two t-curves are compared with the normal. As suggested by the graph, the similarity between the t and normal curves is stronger when r is large. When r is larger than 30, the probability density curve of the t-variable is so close to that of the standard normal that areas under the latter may be used as good approximations to the less extensively tabulated probabilities of Student's t.

For $r = 1$ to 30, and for a few selected larger values of r, Table IV in the Appendix gives values of t corresponding to each specified area P in the right tail of the distribution.

Referring to the table, we see, for instance, that if T has a t-distribution with 10 degrees of freedom, $P(T > 2.764) = 0.01$. Because of the symmetry of the t-distribution, the table can also be read for *negative* values of T that correspond to a given area P in the *left* tail.

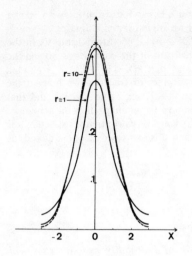

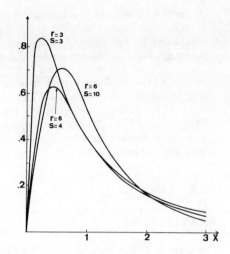

FIG. 4.13. Student's t density curves (solid lines) compared with the standard normal (dotted line).

'FIG. 4.14. F density curves.

4.4 g. The F distribution

If U is a χ^2 variable with r degrees of freedom, and V another χ^2 variable with s degrees of freedom and independent of U, then the ratio

$$F = \frac{U/r}{V/s}$$

has an F distribution with (r , s) degrees of freedom. The two parameters of this distribution are the ordered pair (r , s).

From its definition, it is clear that F cannot be negative and that it can assume indefinitely large positive values. Its mean depends only on the degrees of freedom in the denominator and is equal to $s/(s-2)$. Three different F density curves are shown in Figure 4.14.

Various tables of probabilities for F variables have been constructed. Since each distribution depends on two parameters, it is difficult to provide much information in a table of reasonable size. Table Va in the Appendix gives values of F exceeded with a probability P of 5%, and Table Vb gives values exceeded with a probability of 1%, for a number of combinations of r and s. These are sufficient for use in most applications. Moreover, since an F variable with (r,s) degrees of freedom is the reciprocal of an F variable with (s,r) degrees of freedom, and since $P(F \leqslant c) = P(1/F \geqslant 1/c)$, the tables can also be used to find values corresponding to 5% and 1% areas in the *lower* tail of the distribution, as illustrated in the following example.

Example 4.10. Suppose it is known that a statistic X has an F distribution with 10 and 20 degrees of freedom (r = 10, s = 20), and that we are interested in finding two numbers, a and b, such that $P(X \leqslant a) = .05$ and $P(X \geqslant b) = .05$. From Table Va in the Appendix, we read b as the number at the intersection of the column r = 10 and the row s = 20, so that b = 2.35. To find a, we recall that $P(X \leqslant a) = P(1/X \geqslant 1/a)$ and since 1/X has an F distribution with (20, 10) degrees of freedom, we look at the intersection of the column r = 20 and the row s = 10 in Table Va and find that 1/a = 2.77, therefore a = .36. The two results can now be summarized in the statement $P(.36 < X < 2.77) = .90$, We note in passing that, since F is a continuous variable, it is immaterial whether the interval bounded by a and b is expressed as open, closed, or half-open and half-closed.

REFERENCES

Burington, R.S. and May, D.C. (1970). *Handbook of Probability and Statistics with Tables,* 2nd ed., Handbook Publishers, Sandusky, Ohio, U.S.A.

Cook, R.D. and Nassar, R.F. (1972). Dynamics of finite populations I. The expected time to fixation or loss and the probability of fixation of an allele in a haploid population of variable size. Biometrics, journal of The Biometric Society, *28,* 373-384.

Duncan, I.B. and Curnow, R.N. (1978). Operational research in the health and social Services. Jl R. statist. Soc. *A 141,* 153-194.

Ederer, F., Myers, M.H. and Mantel, N. (1964). A statistical problem in space and time: do leukemia cases come in clusters? Biometrics, journal of The Biometric Society, *20,* 626-638.

Feigl, P. and Zelen, M. (1965). Estimation of exponential survival probabilities with concomitant information. Biometrics, journal of The Biometric Society, *21,* 826-838.

Kendall, M.G. and Stuart, A. (1969). *The Advanced Theory of Statistics,* vol. I, 3rd ed., Charles Griffin & Co., London.

Layard, M.W.J. and Arvesen, J.N. (1978). Analysis of Poisson data in cross-over experimental design. Biometrics, journal of The Biometric Society, *34,* 421-428.

Maritz, J.S. (1957). A model for the deterioration in strength of materials due to fungal attack. Biometrics, journal of The Biometric Society, *13,* 433-441

Mazumdar, M. and Kussmaul, K.L. (1967). A study of the variability due to coincident passage in an electronic blood cell counter. Biometrics, journal of The Biometric Society, *23,* 671-684.

Parratt, L.G. (1961). *Probability and Experimental Errors in Science.* Wiley, New York.

Pearson, E.S. and Hartley, H.O. (editors) (1966). *Biometrika Tables for Statisticans*, vol. I, 3rd ed., Cambridge University Press, Cambridge, England.

Thomas, V.J., Doughty, N.A., Fletcher, R.H., and Robertson, J.G. (1972). Estimation of microbial viability. Biometrics, journal of The Biometric Society, *28*, 947-958.

Uhler, R.S. and Bradley, P.G. (1970). A stochastic model for determining the economic prospects of petroleum exploration over large regions. J.Am. statist. Ass. *65*, 623-630.

CHAPTER 5
Techniques of Statistical Inference

5.1. INTRODUCTION

In this chapter, we consider methods by which sample data can be used to shed some light on unknown properties of the populations sampled. This transition from sample observations to the drawing of conclusions about underlying populations is known as *statistical inference*. Methods of statistical inference applicable to specific types of problems will be taken up in detail in later chapters. Here, the presentation is quite general, being meant to acquaint the reader with a few basic techniques and prepare the ground for their application. Which of the various techniques presented is to be used in any particular problem depends very much on the nature of the information that is being sought, as illustrated by the following hypothetical situations:

(i) It is known that the survival time after diagnosis for a certain condition is a variable whose probability distribution is exponential with an unknown mean μ. If a number of observations on this variable are available, they can be used to calculate an estimate of the population mean. This is a problem in *point estimation*.

(ii) The systolic blood pressure in a certain community is known to be normally distributed with an unknown standard deviation σ. We may use a sample from this population to find boundaries of an interval which, we can be fairly certain, contains the unknown parameter σ. This is a problem in *interval estimation*.

(iii) The rate of recovery following the administration of a drug, call it A, is known to be 65% . A new and more expensive drug, B, will be adopted if we can be fairly sure that it has a recovery rate higher than 65%. On the basis of a sample of observations from the users of drug B, we decide whether or not to adopt it. This is a problem in *hypothesis testing*.

(iv) In a certain age group, it is suspected that the incidence of duodenal ulcer is higher among the more highly educated members of the group. A sample from this population can be used to decide whether or not the two variables, incidence of ulcer and degree of education, are related. This is another problem in *hypothesis testing*.

In all of the above problems, decisions are based on sample observations and statistics calculated therefrom, and therefore on variable quantities that are subject to random fluctuations from sample to sample. These random fluctuations, which are best described in terms of the sampling distributions of the statistics used, are taken into account in all the methods of statistical inference outlined in this chapter.

Making inferences about a population is not always an end in itself. Information obtained through statistical inference can be used in making *predictions* for future observations. One such use will be illustrated in Section 14.3.

5.2. POINT ESTIMATION

To estimate an unknown parameter of a population is to find a number that is believed to be very close to the unknown quantity. This number is usually obtained from a representative sample, and is therefore the value of a statistic. In this book, we shall refer to both the estimating statistic and to its numerical value as *"estimate"* and, following conventional usage, we shall denote the estimate of a parameter θ (theta) by the corresponding symbol $\hat{\theta}$ (theta hat). θ might be the mean of a Poisson variable, the proportion of a bionomial variable, the standard deviation of a normal variable, etc.

In choosing appropriate statistics to use as estimates of the various parameters, statisticians have been guided by a number of principles, outstanding among which are the following:

(i) The estimate must be *unbiased* in the sense that its distribution is centered at the unknown parameter. More precisely, $\hat{\theta}$ is an unbiased estimate of θ if $E(\hat{\theta}) = \theta$. This requirement insures that the particular method of calculating the estimate $\hat{\theta}$ is correct "on the average".

(ii) The estimate must also be *as precise as possible*. In terms of the sampling distribution of $\hat{\theta}$, we require that the standard deviation of $\hat{\theta}$ — or its *standard error*, as it is also called — be as small as possible. This requirement insures that the estimate is the most reliable of the unbiased estimates.

Wherever possible in the following chapters, we shall use point estimates that are known to be unbiased and most precise. In most cases, the estimates will also turn out to be those statistics that would have seemed appropriate for estimation on a purely intuitive basis.

An indication of the reliability of an estimate is often stated in terms of its standard error (S.E.) or, if that is unknown, by an estimate thereof. This often appears in the literature in the form: (a number) ± (another number), which is to be read as: $\hat{\theta}$ ± estimated S.E.$(\hat{\theta})$.

Once an estimate for a parameter has been found, it can be used to estimate any quantity whose value depends on that unknown parameter, that is, any function of the parameter. For example, to estimate the probability, say P, that an exponential variable with unknown mean exceeds a given number c, which is $P = e^{-c/\mu}$, we replace the unknown μ by its estimate to obtain $\hat{P} = e^{-c/\hat{\mu}}$. It must be pointed out, however, that such substitutions do not in general yield optimum estimates of the functions, for although $\hat{\mu}$ may be the most precise unbiased estimate of μ, $\hat{P} = e^{-c/\hat{\mu}}$ is a biased estimate of P.

5.3. CONSTRUCTING CONFIDENCE INTERVALS

A confidence interval for a parameter θ is defined in terms of two statistics, S_1 and

S_2 (where $S_1 < S_2$), which are believed to fall on either side of the unknown θ, or that

$$S_1 \leqslant \theta \leqslant S_2.$$

Interval estimation goes a step beyond point estimation by providing, in addition to the estimating interval (S_1, S_2), a measure of one's confidence in the correctness of the estimate. This measure is given by the probability C that the interval does in fact contain the fixed point θ, or $C = P(S_1 \leqslant \theta \leqslant S_2)$. The interval (S_1, S_2) is called the *confidence interval*, S_1 and S_2 are the lower and upper *confidence limits*, and the probability C is known as the *confidence level* or *confidence coefficient*.

Constructing a confidence interval is like performing a single trial in a game of chance in which the outcome is success if the confidence limits happen to straddle the fixed point θ and failure if the interval completely misses that point. Whether the outcome is success or failure depends, therefore, on the numerical values of S_1 and S_2 which vary from sample to sample, and hence on the composition of the sample. The confidence coefficient, which is the probability of success, can then be interpreted as the proportion of all the possible confidence intervals, each drawn from a different possible sample, that contain the parameter θ.

It will be seen in the specific applications of this technique to particular parameters that the statistics S_1 and S_2 are usually functions of the point estimate $\hat{\theta}$. In each case, the particular functions are such that C can be determined from the sampling distribution of $\hat{\theta}$. In practice, however, rather than set up an interval and determine its confidence level, we assign a value to C depending upon the desired confidence, and then determine the limits S_1 and S_2 corresponding to it.

5.4. TESTING OF STATISTICAL HYPOTHESES

When a population parameter θ is completely unknown, it may be estimated by the methods of the two previous sections. But there are situations in which, although θ is unknown, one may have reasons to suspect it to have some specific value, say k. In such a case, one postulates a hypothesis in which it is stated that $\theta = k$; then, on the basis of a set of observations from the population being considered, one decides whether to accept or reject that hypothesis. The manner in which the sample observations are used to reach this decision is called the *test* of the *statistical hypothesis* that $\theta = k$.

Statistical hypotheses are not necessarily restricted to statements about parameter values. A variety of problems that can be formulated as statistical hypotheses will be encountered in chapters 6 to 16 and the appropriate test will be described in each case. A few examples of statistical hypotheses are listed here for illustration:

(i) The hypothesis that a variable, like gain in weight, has a certain stated distribution such as the normal. This is a hypothesis on the validity of a statistical model.

(ii) The hypothesis that two different sets of observations, like gain in weight under diet A and gain in weight under diet B, come from populations with equal means. This is a hypothesis that is very commonly used in comparative studies.

(iii) A hypothesis that two variables observed simultaneously, such as color of eyes and color of hair, are not associated. This is a hypothesis of independence between two variables.

As the above examples suggest, a statistical hypothesis is a statement about the distributions of the observed variables in their populations. Usually, the statement is one in which a claim is denied, such as: there is *no* difference between the two means, there is *no* relation between the two variables, there is *no* change in the value of the parameter since the population was last observed, there is *no* discrepancy between the model and the population, etc. For this reason, the hypothesis being tested is often referred to as the *null hypothesis.* We shall use the terms "hypothesis tested" and "null hypothesis" interchangeably.

Hypothesis testing involves the following steps:

1) Once the problem is identified, a null hypothesis is stated. This hypothesis is denoted by H_0.

2) A random sample is taken from the population (or populations) with which H_0 is concerned.

3) A statistic (or more than one statistic) is calculated from the sample. The decision to accept or reject H_0 will be based on the value of this statistic, which is therefore called the *test statistic.*

4) By an inspection of the sampling distribution of the test statistic when the null hypothesis is true, some values of the statistic are judged unlikely to occur under the assumptions of H_0 (and hence their occurrence would cast doubt on its validity). These are called *significant values* of the test statistic. They usually lie in the tails of its sampling distribution and are determined by the condition that their probability of occurrence under H_0 is no more than a preassigned small number, α, known as the *significance level* of the test.

5) The calculated value of the test statistic (step (3)) is compared with the set of significant values corresponding to a given significance level α (step (4)). If the value of the statistic belongs to this set, it is pronounced *significant at level α*, and the null hypothesis is rejected. Otherwise, H_0 is accepted. This rule constitutes the test of H_0 at level α.

A few remarks will now be made in connection with this outline of the testing procedure.

(i) Rejecting a null hypothesis does not mean that it is not true, but simply that the particular sample observed does not support it. In fact, it is understood that significant values of the test statistic *can* occur when H_0 is true, the probability of their occurring (and therefore the probability that H_0 is rejected while true) being no more than the significance level α. α is thus an upper limit for the probability that an error is committed by rejecting a true hypothesis. The rejection of a true hypothesis is called an *error of Type I.*

(ii) Since α is a ceiling on the probability of an error in decision, it is usually taken to be a small number, 1% and 5% being the most commonly used significance levels*. But although a small α is desirable, it makes no sense to make it zero, as that would imply that no values of the test statistic would be significant, and that H_0 would be accepted whatever the sample observations might be.

(iii) There is implicit in the rejection of a null hypothesis the supposition that some alternative theory may provide a better description of the population than the one given

---

* These two levels occur so frequently in applications that a special notation has evolved and often appears in tabulated results in the literature. In this notation, the calculated value of the test statistic followed by one asterisk (*) denotes significance at the 5% level, and the calculated value followed by two asterisks (**) denotes significance at the 1% level.

by H_0. Frequently, this is provided for in the formulation of the problem, where both a null hypothesis H_0 and an *alternative hypothesis* are stated, and the purpose is to test H_0 against that alternative. In this case, a rejection of H_0 is equivalent to an acceptance of the alternative hypothesis, and vice versa.

(iv) When an alternative hypothesis is specified in addition to the hypothesis tested, this is taken into account in delineating the significant values of the test statistic. These values must be unlikely when the hypothesis tested is true but quite likely when the alternative is true, since their occurrence is taken as evidence in favor of the latter. For example, if the sampling distributions of the test statistic under the null hypothesis H_0 and the alternative hypothesis H_R are as shown in Figure 5.1(a), only large values of the statistic are considered significant. If, on the other hand, H_0 is tested against H_L, as shown in Figure 5.1(b), only small values of the statistic are considered significant.

(a)   (b)

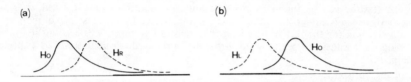

FIG. 5.1 Sampling distributions of a test statistic under two different hypotheses.
Significant values of the statistic are marked by a heavy line.

(v) It is quite possible for a null hypothesis to be accepted while the alternative hypothesis is the true one. This can happen when the alternative hypothesis is true and yet the test statistic, purely by chance, assumes values that are not unlikely under H_0 and therefore not considered significant. Accepting a false hypothesis is called an *error of Type II*. The probability of such an error can be calculated if the distribution of the test statistic under the alternative is completely specified.

(vi) We note that P(error of Type I), being less than or equal to the preassigned level of significance, can be kept arbitrarily small. P(error of Type II), on the other hand, depends on the values of the test statistic that are considered significant, and this probability may turn out to be uncomfortably large. In view of this, when two conflicting hypotheses are to be tested against each other, it is advisable to *take as H_0 that hypothesis whose rejection when true would be the more serious of the two errors*.

(vii) Instead of fixing a significance level and then judging the sample outcome as significant or not at that level, some investigators prefer to calculate what is called the *P-value* of the sample. The P-value is the probability that, if the hypothesis tested is true, the test statistic can assume values equal to or more extreme (and, as such, less likely) than the one actually calculated. The smaller the P-value, the less support the sample is seen to give to the hypothesis tested. Clearly, if the hypothesis is rejected at level α, the P-value of the test statistic must be α or less.

(viii) If a hypothesis about the distribution of a variable does not specify the distribution uniquely, it is called a *composite* hypothesis. For example, the null hypothesis

$$H_0 : \mu \leqslant k$$

where μ is the mean of a Poisson variable and k is a constant, is composite. Any value of μ that does not exceed k is a possible mean for X under this hypothesis, and each μ characterizes a different distribution for X. A possible alternative hypothesis to H_0 is

$$H_R : \mu > k$$

which is also composite. We note that there must be no overlap between the two sets of values of μ allowed by a null hypothesis and its alternative.

When a hypothesis is not composite, it is called *simple*. Either the hypothesis tested or the alternative hypothesis may be simple or composite. Thus one may test H_0 as defined above against $H_R : \mu = |k| + 1$, which is simple, or one can test the simple hypothesis $H_0 : \mu = k$ against the composite alternative $H_R : \mu > k$, etc.

As long as the hypothesis tested is simple, the test can be carried out in the usual way (whether the alternative hypothesis is simple or composite), since the significant values of the test statistic can be found from its (unique) distribution under H_0. But when the hypothesis tested is composite, the problem is complicated by the existence of more than one distribution for the test statistic and they must all be taken into account in finding the significant values. To see how this difficulty is resolved, we refer again to a specific example: −

For the Poisson variable with mean μ, suppose that we wish to test $H_0 : \mu \leqslant k$ against $H_R : \mu > k$ on the basis of one observation X, at a level of significance α. It is easy to see in this example that large values of X, say $X > r$, should lead to a rejection of H_0 and small values to its acceptance. The problem is to find a suitable r to satisfy the condition that the level of significance is α; that is, r must be chosen in such a way that the probability P(error of Type I), which is the same as $P(X > r)$ when H_0 is true, is less than or equal to α for *all* distributions having $\mu \leqslant k$. This is accomplished by making $P(X > r)$ *equal* to α for the distribution in H_0 that is *closest* to those in H_R, namely the distribution in which $\mu = k$. This choice of r brings about the desired results because, if the probability $P(X > r)$ is α when $\mu = k$, it must be smaller than α when the entire distribution is shifted to lower values of X, that is, when $\mu < k$.

CHAPTER 6
The Proportion of
a Qualitative Variable

6.1. INTRODUCTION

When observations are made on a qualitative variable, there are in general several categories into which an observation may be classified. Frequently, however, interest is focussed on one special category, and each observation on the variable is classified as either belonging to that category or falling outside it. Thus only two categories are recognized for such a variable, and the variable is called *dichotomous* With a dichotomous variable, the problem is one of finding out what proportion in the population belong to the special category. Questions like the following are fairly common: what proportion of births in a certain year are male births? What proportion of the patients undergoing certain therapy recover completely? What proportion of the instruments obtained from a certain manufacturer are faulty? ... In each case, the population proportion is an unknown parameter, which we shall call p.

In this chapter, the methods of statistical inference introduced in Chapter 5 will be applied to the problem of the unknown parameter p. A random sample of size n will be assumed to have been drawn from the population in question and it will be assumed that the number of sample elements belonging to the special category has been counted.

6.2. CALCULATION OF THE POINT ESTIMATE

Suppose that in the sample of size n exactly X elements are found to belong to the special category. Then a reasonable estimate of the population proportion is the sample proportion X/n. That is,

$$\hat{p} = X/n. \tag{6.1}$$

This is an unbiased estimate. Its standard error is S.E.$(\hat{p}) = \sqrt{p(1-p)/n}$. However, since p is unknown, we use the

$$\text{estimated S.E.}(\hat{p}) = \sqrt{X(n-X)/n^3}. \tag{6.2}$$

These calculations can easily be carried out on a small calculator.

Note: If sampling is done *without replacement* from a small population, the proportions of the two categories are changed with the drawing of each observation, and this change is reflected in the sampling distribution of the statistic p̂. As a result, the standard error of p̂ is diminished by a factor which depends on the relative sizes of the population and sample, and which may be ignored if the *sampling fraction,* or ratio of sample to population size, is less than 10%. In general, in sampling without replacement,

$$\text{S.E.}(\hat{p}) = \sqrt{\frac{p(1-p)}{n} \cdot \frac{N-n}{N-1}} \; .$$

where N is the population size. The factor $(N-n)/(N-1)$ is called the *finite population correction.*

> *Example 6.1* In the hypothetical sample of Example 3.1 (and in Table 3.1), 31 of the 60 births were male. Thus $n = 60$, $X = 31$, and p is estimated as $\hat{p} = .517$, with an estimated standard error of $\sqrt{(31)(29)/60^3} = .065$.

6.3. SAMPLING DISTRIBUTION OF THE ESTIMATE

The statistic X used in estimating p is readily recognized as having a binomial distribution with parameters n and p (Section 4.4. a) and an approximately normal distribution when n is large (Section 4.4 c). Since X has mean np and standard deviation $\sqrt{np(1-p)}$, the standardized variable $Z = (X-np)/\sqrt{np(1-p)}$ is approximately standard normal and, after dividing its numerator and denominator by n, so is

$$Z = \frac{\hat{p}-p}{\sqrt{p(1-p)/n}} \; .$$

(It will be recalled from Section 4.4 c that the approximation is reasonably good when both np and $n(1-p)$ are at least equal to 5.) This distribution has been used in deriving the approximate confidence intervals and tests of hypotheses about p which will be given in the next two sections.

6.4. CONFIDENCE INTERVALS

6.4 a. Exact Confidence Intervals. These are based on the exact distribution of p̂ and, for selected confidence levels, the confidence limits can be read from special charts, such as the ones given in Pearson and Hartley (1966,Table 41), which give intervals corresponding to the 95% and 99% confidence levels. These charts are used when n is so small that the normal approximation to the binomial distribution is considered unreliable. To check on whether a sample is large enough, we apply a modified form of the rule given in Section 4.4 c: If neither np̂ nor $n(1-\hat{p})$ is less than 5, we may feel justified in using the normal approximation and drawing conclusions based on an approximate confidence interval.

A numerical comparison between exact and approximate confidence intervals for a few illustrative cases will be shown in Table 6.1.

6.4 b. Approximate Confidence Intervals.

These are based on the normal approximation.   Denote the desired level of confidence by $1 - \alpha$, and let $z(\alpha/2)$ be the percentile of the standard normal variable Z satisfying the condition $P(-z(\alpha/2) < Z < z(\alpha/2)) = 1-\alpha$. With this notation, the limits of the confidence interval for p at level $1-\alpha$ are given by

$$\hat{p} \pm (z(\alpha/2)\sqrt{\hat{p}(1-\hat{p})/n + 1/2n}), \tag{6.3}$$

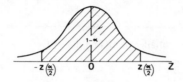

FIG. 6.1.   Two percentiles of the standard normal distribution

where $\hat{p}$ is the estimate defined in Equation (6.1). The term $1/2n$ is the "correction for continuity" and may be ignored when n is very large.   Approximate confidence intervals for p at 90, 95 or 99 percent confidence levels can also be obtained by means of Program PROP1 of Chapter 18.

In reporting confidence limits as in (6.3), one must also state the level at which those limits were obtained. This has the advantage of making the interval more informative and distinguishes confidence intervals from intervals of the type: estimate ± S.E. (estimate), which frequently appear in the literature. The similarity between these two forms is not accidental, since the interval $\hat{p} \pm$ estimated S.E. $(\hat{p})$ coincides with the confidence interval (6.3) in which $z(\alpha/2)$ is equal to 1. It can be easily verified that for such an interval $1-\alpha$ is approximately 68%.

Example 6.2 Abou-Daoud (1969) has recorded the systolic and diastolic blood pressures of full-time employees at the American University of Beirut in the academic year 1967-68. In a random sample of 106 employees, 5 were found to suffer from hypertension. We wish to find a 95% confidence interval for the proportion of the individuals in the population with hypertension. From the sample, we have n = 106, X = 5 and, from the normal distribution table, we find that z(.025) = 1.96. Substituting these values in Formula (6.3), we obtain .047 ± .045 or the interval (.002, .092) as the 95% confidence interval for p.

The following table gives a numerical comparison of exact and approximate confidence intervals in some arbitrarily selected data sets. The exact intervals were obtained from the charts referred to in Section 6.4 a above, while the approximate intervals were calculated from Formula (6.3). In all cases, the smaller of the two numbers, $n\hat{p}$ and $n(1-\hat{p})$, was no less than 5; we remark that the approximation appears distinctly better with larger values of this criterion.

Table 6.1. A comparison of 95% confidence intervals obtained by exact and approximate methods

Sample Characteristics			Exact interval	Approximate interval
n	X	Min*		
10	5	5	(.19, .82)	(.14, .86)
20	8	8	(.19, .64)	(.16, .64)
40	26	14	(.48, .79)	(.48, .79)
100	70	30	(.60, .80)	(.60, .80)

* "Min" stands for the smaller of $n\hat{p}$ and $n(1-\hat{p})$.

6.4 c. Sample Size

Formula (6.3) reveals an important feature of the confidence interval for p, namely that — other things being equal — a larger sample results in a shorter interval, and hence in a more precise estimate of p. While this is not surprising in itself, it is useful for finding the sample size required to achieve a prescribed degree of precision. This will be shown in the following discussion where, to simplify the formulas, we drop the correction for continuity, assuming that the samples under discussion have sufficiently large sizes to justify doing so.

We first observe that the $1-\alpha$ confidence interval for p can be expressed in the form

$$\hat{p} - z(\alpha/2)\sqrt{\hat{p}(1-\hat{p})/n} \leq p \leq \hat{p} + z(\alpha/2)\sqrt{\hat{p}(1-\hat{p})/n}$$

or, more briefly, in the form

$$|\hat{p} - p| \leq z(\alpha/2)\sqrt{\hat{p}(1-\hat{p})/n},$$

which shows that, with probability $1-\alpha$, the estimate $\hat{p}$ is within $z(\alpha/2)\sqrt{\hat{p}(1-\hat{p})/n}$ units of p. This quantity is a variable that depends on $\hat{p}$, a matter which should detract from its value as a measure of the precision of $\hat{p}$. However, since the product of a fraction and its complement cannot exceed 1/4, $\hat{p}(1-\hat{p})/n \leq 1/4n$, and therefore the maximum discrepancy between p and $\hat{p}$, which is $z(\alpha/2)\sqrt{\hat{p}(1-\hat{p})/n}$, is no more than $z(\alpha/2)/2\sqrt{n}$, no matter what $\hat{p}$ may be.

If we now wish to estimate p at level $1-\alpha$ to within d units of its true value (where d is an arbitrary number between 0 and 1), regardless of what $\hat{p}$ may turn out to be, we must take a sample of size n that satisfies the condition $z(\alpha/2)/2\sqrt{n} \leq d$, or

$$n \geq \left(\frac{z(\alpha/2)}{2d}\right)^2. \tag{6.4}$$

6.5. HYPOTHESIS TESTING

A hypothesis about the proportion in a dichotomous population is a statement about the value of the parameter p. We shall consider in this section the problem of testing the simple hypothesis $H_0 : p = p_0$, where p_0 is a specified number, against different types of alternatives. The tests of H_0 will also be found appropriate for a number of composite null hypotheses related to H_0.

The test statistic is the number of elements in the sample belonging to the special category. This is denoted by X, whose sampling distribution was given in Section 6.3. In the following presentation, the sample size n will be assumed large enough to permit the use of the normal approximation as the sampling distribution. The small-sample case will be commented upon at the end of the section.

Since X is approximately normally distributed with mean np and standard deviation $\sqrt{np(1-p)}$, the standardized variable

$$Z = \frac{X-np}{\sqrt{np(1-p)}}$$

has approximately the standard normal distribution. Instead of expressing the test in terms of significant values of X, we shall find it more convenient to express it in terms of the corresponding significant values of Z. The correction for continuity will appear as half a unit added to or subtracted from X.

We take α as the significance level for each of the following tests, and we use $z(\alpha)$ to denote the $100(1-\alpha)$ percentile of the standard normal distribution, or the value of Z that is exceeded with probability α (see Figure 6.1). We distinguish three types of testing situations, depending on the nature of the alternative hypothesis. For the sake of generality, the latter will be taken as composite.

(i) $H_0 : p = p_0$ against $H_R : p > p_0$
   or $H'_0 : p \leqslant p_0$ against $H_R : p > p_0$

These alternatives are *right-sided*. Since the mean of the sampling distribution of the statistic X is np, X tends on the average to be larger under H_R than under H_0 or H'_0, and the significant values are therefore *in the right tail* of its distribution under H_0, as in Figure 6.2(a). The significant values are given by

$$\frac{X-np_0 - \frac{1}{2}}{\sqrt{np_0(1-p_0)}} > z(\alpha) . \tag{6.5}$$

(ii) $H_0 : p = p_0$ against $H_L : p < p_0$
   or $H'_0 : p \geqslant p_0$ against $H_L : p < p_0$

These are *left-sided* alternatives, and by analogy with case (a) we see that the significant values of X must be *in the left tail* of its distribution under H_0, as in Figure 6.2(b). The significant values are given by

$$\frac{X - np_0 + \frac{1}{2}}{\sqrt{np_0(1-p_0)}} < -z(\alpha). \tag{6.6}$$

(iii) $H_0 : p = p_0$ against $H_T : p \neq p_0$

Since the alternative hypothesis is *two-sided*, the significant values of X are *in the two tails* of its distribution under H_0, as in Figure 6.2(c). The significant values are given by

$$\frac{X-np_0 - \frac{1}{2}}{\sqrt{np_0\,(1-p_0)}} > z(\alpha/2) \text{ in the right tail, and}$$

$$\frac{X-np_0 + \frac{1}{2}}{\sqrt{np_0\,(1-p_0)}} < -z(\alpha/2) \text{ in the left tail.}$$

These two can be summarized in the more convenient form

$$\frac{|X-np_0| - \frac{1}{2}}{\sqrt{np_0\,(1-p_0)}} > z(\alpha/2). \tag{6.7}$$

The standardized variable for each of the above tests may be obtained by means of Program PROP2 of Chapter 18.

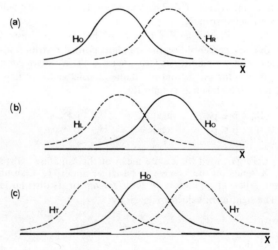

FIG. 6.2. Testing against (a) right-sided, (b) left-sided, and (c) two-sided
alternatives (significant values of test statistic are denoted by a heavy line)

Example 6.3.   A batch of 100 mg tablets is to be inspected for uniformity in weight. If more than 10% of the tablets deviate from the prescribed weight of 100 mgs by more than an acceptable margin, the batch will be considered not within the pharmacopoeia limit specifications and returned to the supplier. We assume that the decision will be taken after a careful weighing of a random sample of 50 tablets taken from this batch. If 8 out of this sample of 50 are found to have weights outside the margin, what decision should be taken on the entire batch?

Here $n = 50$, $X = 8$, $H_0 : p \leqslant .10$ and $H_R : p > .10$, so that $p_0 = .10$. Take α as 1%, then $z(.01) = 2.33$. Applying (6.5), we calculate the standardized X as

$$\frac{8-5-.5}{\sqrt{4.5}} = 1.18$$

and compare it with 2.33. Since it is not larger than 2.33, we accept H_0 and retain the batch of tablets.

The P-value of the observed X is $P(Z > 1.18)$. Referring to Table II in the Appendix, we find this probability to be 0.12.

To calculate the probability of an error of Type II (that is, the probability of accepting a false hypothesis) when the value of p is .15, we proceed as follows: find the non-significant values of X given by the test, standardize those values using $p = .15$, and calculate their probability. Thus the probability

$$P \text{ (Error of Type II)} = P(\frac{X-5.5}{\sqrt{4.5}} \leqslant 2.33) \text{ when p } = .15$$

$$= P(X \leqslant 10.44) \text{ when p } = .15$$

$$= P(Z \leqslant \frac{10.44-7.50-.5}{2.52})$$

since, when $p = .15$, $np = 7.50$ and $\sqrt{np(1-p)} = 2.52$,

$$= P(Z \leqslant 0.97) = .8340.$$

The risk of accepting a batch containing a proportion of 15% that are outside the limits is therefore 83.4%

If the sample is small, the exact sampling distribution of X (which is binomial) should be used in the testing procedure. Since the binomial distribution is discrete with each integer X carrying a non-zero probability, it may be impossible to find a set of significant values of X corresponding exactly to a preassigned level α. In this case, it is simpler to calculate the P-value of the observed X. Let the observed value of X be c. Then the P-value is calculated as:

$P(X \geqslant c)$ in testing against a right-sided alternative,
$P(X \leqslant c)$ in testing against a left-sided alternative, and
$P(X \geqslant c) + P(X \leqslant 2np_0 - c)$ if $c > np_0$ and the alternative is 2-sided, or
$P(X \leqslant c) + P(X \geqslant 2np_0 - c)$ if $c < np_0$ and the alternative is 2-sided.

The probabilities in all these cases are obtained by Program PROB2 of Chapter 18 or from tables of the binomial distribution (Burington and May, 1970) with the given n and $p = p_0$.

REFERENCES

Abou-Daoud, K.T. (1969). Blood pressure, height and weight status of a group of Lebanese. J. med. liban, *22*, 591-601.

Burington, R.S. and May, D.C. (1970). *Handbook of Probability and Statistics With Tables,* 2nd ed., Handbook Publishers, Sandusky, Ohio, U.S.A.

Pearson, E.S. and Hartley, H.O. (editors) (1966). *Biometrika Tables for Statisticians,* vol. I, 3rd ed., Cambridge University Press, Cambridge, England.

CHAPTER 7
The Standard Deviation of a Numerical Variable

7.1. INTRODUCTION

When the observed variable is numerical, one of the characteristics of its probability distribution that we may wish to investigate is the degree of variability inherent in that distribution. For example, a measurement may be known to fluctuate from reading to reading on the same instrument, and in order to gauge the reliability of a single observation we need some information on the amount of fluctuation involved in such measurements. Or, while under normal conditions individuals may be expected to vary from a "standard" in their responses to a certain stimulus, it is necessary to know just how much variation can be attributed to chance alone before the response of a single individual is judged normal or not.

Of the three measures of variability (or dispersion) considered in Section 4.3, the most commonly used is the standard deviation σ, to which we shall confine our attention in this chapter. The reasons for this preference for σ as a measure of dispersion are theoretical. With it as the parameter, the problems of estimation and hypothesis testing are considerably simplified, particularly when the sample is taken from a normal population, as is frequently the case with numerical observations. We shall find it easier to formulate the problem in terms of the variance σ^2, which is defined as $\sigma^2 = \Sigma (x-\mu)^2 \cdot P(X = x)$ when X is discrete. Since σ cannot be negative, any conclusion about σ^2 can immediately be translated without ambiguity into a conclusion about σ.

7.2. CALCULATION OF THE ESTIMATE

7.2 a. Raw Data

Suppose that a sample of size n has been taken from a population whose standard deviation is σ. Denote the sample observations by $X_1, \ldots, X_n$ and their arithmetical average by $\overline{X}$. Then an unbiased estimate of the population variance σ^2 is the sample variance

$$\hat{\sigma}^2 = s^2 = \sum_{i=1}^{n} (X_i - \overline{X})^2 / (n-1) . \tag{7.1}$$

We notice from Equation (7.1) that, had its denominator been n instead of n−1, the estimate s^2 would have been strictly analogous to σ^2 in being a weighted sum of the squared deviations of the variables from their mean. Division of the sum of squares by $n-1$ has the advantage of making the estimate unbiased. Moreover, $n-1$ is the correct count of the *degrees of freedom*, or the number of quantities that are free to vary, in the numerator of s^2. This number is $n-1$ because the n deviations $X_i-\overline{X}$ are subject to one restriction, namely that their sum must be zero; because of this restriction, if $n-1$ of the deviations are given, the nth is also known, as it must be the difference between zero and the sum of the others. In general, if n variables are subject to r different restrictions, the degrees of freedom of the set of variables is reduced from n to $n-r$.

Although the form of Equation (7.1) is appropriate for defining s^2, it is cumbersome to use in calculations. By a simple algebraic manipulation of this equation, we can easily arrive at the computational form,

$$s^2 = \frac{\Sigma\, X_i^2 - (\Sigma\, X_i\,)^2\, /\, n}{n-1}\,, \tag{7.2}$$

where the summation is for $i = 1$ to $i = n$. This calls for little more than the calculation of the statistics ΣX_i and ΣX_i^2, both of which can be obtained on a simple desk or pocket calculator. Some calculators are also equipped with special function keys which include s or s^2, in which case only the data set $X_1, \ldots, X_n$ is needed. Alternatively, s^2 and s may be read from the output of Program DESC2 of Chapter 18.

Note (1). Although the sample variance s^2 is an unbiased estimate of the population variance σ^2, the standard deviation s tends to slightly underestimate σ, particularly in very small samples. The larger the sample is, the more negligible is this bias and the closer to σ is s likely to be.

Note (2). It can be shown that the statistic s^2 remains unchanged if a constant is added to or subtracted from each observation; that is, s^2 is *invariant* under a change of origin. To see this, we note that if each X_i is replaced by $X_i + c$ (where c is any constant) then $\overline{X}$ is also replaced by $\overline{X} + c$. Thus each difference $X_i-\overline{X}$ remains unchanged, and so does the numerator in Equation (7.1). This invariance property sometimes reduces the labor of calculations considerably. But it must be pointed out that this property does not hold for all statistics that one may want to calculate from the same sample.

Note (3). In normal samples, a quick and unbiased estimate of σ can be obtained from the sample range, which is the difference between the largest and the smallest sample observations, and which is easily determined in a small or even moderately large sample by inspection. The estimate, based on the sampling distribution of the sample range, is obtained by multiplying the sample range by a factor, call it f_n, which depends on the sample size n, and which is given in Table 7.1 for a number of different sample sizes; that is, $\hat{\sigma} = f_n \cdot$ (sample range). This estimate is particularly good when the sample is small.

Table 7.1. Factor for estimating σ from the sample range

Sample Size n	Factor f_n	Sample Size n	Factor f_n
2	0.8862	30	0.2448
3	.5908	35	.2373
4	.4857	40	.2314
5	.4299	45	.2265
6	.3946	50	.2223
7	.3698	55	.2187
8	.3512	60	.2156
9	.3367	65	.2128
10	.3249	70	.2103
11	.3152	75	.2081
12	.3069	80	.2060
13	.2998	85	.2042
14	.2935	90	.2025
15	.2880	95	.2009
16	.2831	100	.1994
17	.2787	200	.1821
18	.2747	300	.1737
19	.2711	400	.1685
20	.2677	500	.1647

Source : Pearson and Hartley (1966, Tables 22 and 27)

Example 7.1. As part of a larger investigation of the water supplies in Lebanon, Acra (1975) has determined the chemical content (in mg/liter) of samples of water taken from a number of different localities in the country. The calcium content of a randomly selected set of 51 water samples originating in the Bekaa and South Lebanon regions is used here to illustrate the calculations of the estimates. The observations, to the nearest mg, were:

68 60 48 84 88   68 76 52 52 64 60 64 56 52 72   56 32

60 48 40 52 64 100 52 64 48 68 76 80 92 56 96 72 28

85 88 40 60 52   84 76 64 92 44 36 44 92 48 36   52 68

From this data, we calculate ΣX_i = 3209 and ΣX_i^2 = 217929. Hence, by (7.2), s^2 = 320.2737 and s = 17.90. By the short-cut method, using the factor corresponding to n = 50 in Table 7.1, we find f_n = .2223 and the sample range 100-28 = 72; hence this estimate of σ is (.2223) (72) = 16.01.

7.2 b. Grouped Data

Suppose that the sample observations have been classified in a frequency distribution with k classes. Let the frequency in the i th class be denoted by f_i and the midpoint of the ith class interval by X_i. Then the appropriate formula for calculating the sample variance, which is equivalent to Equation (7.2), is

$$s^2 = \frac{\Sigma f_i X_i^2 - (\Sigma f_i X_i)^2 / n}{n - 1} \qquad (7.3)$$

where the summation is for $i = 1$ to $i = k$. Alternatively, one can use Program DESC3 of Chapter 18. Because of the loss of information involved in the grouping, this estimate does not have precisely the same value as the one calculated from the raw data.

Example 7.2. A classification of the data of Example 7.1 in a frequency distribution of 9 classes is shown below along with the calculations necessary for the application of Formula (7.3).

i	Class Interval	X_i	f_i	$f_i X_i$	X_i^2	$f_i X_i^2$
1	20 — 30⁻	25	1	25	625	625
2	30 — 40⁻	35	3	105	1225	3675
3	40 — 50⁻	48	8	360	2025	16200
4	50 — 60⁻	55	10	550	3025	30250
5	60 — 70⁻	65	13	845	4225	54925
6	70 — 80⁻	75	5	375	5625	28125
7	80 — 90⁻	85	6	510	7225	43350
8	90 — 100⁻	95	4	380	9025	36100
9	100 — 110⁻	105	1	105	11025	11025
			51	3255		224275

Substituting in (7.3), we get $s^2 = 330.59$, and $s = 18.18$, which is larger than the value obtained before grouping. This is typical of the way grouping inflates the estimate of σ, particularly when the class intervals are wide.

7.2 c. Standard Error of the Estimate

If the variable X has a normal distribution, the standard error of the sample variance is

$$\text{S.E. } (s^2) = \sigma^2 \sqrt{2/(n-1)} \qquad (7.4)$$

which is smaller for larger samples. For practical purposes, since σ is unknown, an estimate of the standard error is calculated from Equation (7.4) with σ replaced by s.

When X is not normal, s^2, while still an unbiassed estimate of σ^2, has a standard error which depends on a characteristic of the distribution known as the "fourth moment" in addition to its dependence on σ. This dependence can be conveniently expressed in terms of a quantity, called *kurtosis*, which is related to both the fourth moment and σ, and is zero in the case of the normal distribution. If we denote the kurtosis of the distribution by K, we can write the standard error of s^2 in the more general form

$$\text{S.E.}(s^2) = \sigma^2 |\sqrt{2/(n-1) + K/n}, \tag{7.5}$$

which shows it to be a larger multiple of σ^2 than in the normal case when K is positive and a smaller multiple when K is negative ($K \geqslant -2n/(n-1)$). Although the kurtosis in a distribution can be estimated from the sample, the calculations are cumbersome. Computer programs which provide a listing of the "descriptive statistics" of a sample usually include an estimate of kurtosis, which can then be used in evaluating the standard error of s^2 in a non-normal sample.

7.3. SAMPLING DISTRIBUTION OF THE ESTIMATE

The estimate s^2 has a well-defined sampling distribution when the sample is drawn from a normal population. In this case, the quantity $(n-1)s^2/\sigma^2$ is distributed as a Chi-square variable with $n-1$ degrees of freedom.

When the parent population is not normal, the sampling distribution of s^2 is not known, and the Chi-square distribution does not provide a good approximation unless the departure from normality is mild. Since the methods of interval estimation and hypothesis testing must utilize the sampling distribution of the statistic, it will be assumed in the next two sections that the samples we are dealing with are normal samples.

7.4. CONFIDENCE INTERVALS

To construct a confidence interval for σ^2 at level $1-\alpha$, we note that, if Y is a Chi-square variable with $n-1$ degrees of freedom, Table III in the Appendix can be used to find two percentiles of the distribution that cut off equal areas in the two tails and contain between them the specified probability, $1-\alpha^*$. Since the total area under the curve is 1, the area in each tail must be $\alpha/2$. These percentiles are shown in Figure 7.1, where $\chi^2_{n-1}(\alpha/2)$ denotes the value of the variable Y that is exceeded with probability $\alpha/2$, and similarly for the other percentile.

---

* It is customary to divide the residual probability α equally between the two tails of the distribution. This division, which often results in the shortest intervals, will be used in future chapters as well.

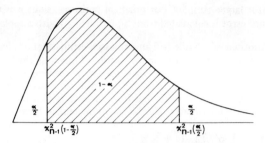

FIG. 7.1.   Two percentiles of a Chi-square distribution

Since $(n-1)s^2/\sigma^2$ has this distribution, $1-\alpha$ is the probability of the event

$$\chi^2_{n-1}(1-\alpha/2) \leqslant (n-1)s^2 \ / \ \sigma^2 \leqslant \chi^2_{n-1}(\alpha/2)$$

which is the same as the event

$$(n-1)s^2 \ /\chi^2_{n-1}(\alpha/2) \leqslant \sigma^2 \leqslant (n-1)s^2 \ /\chi^2_{n-1}(1-\alpha/2), \qquad (7.6)$$

and the two limits of this inequality are the $1-\alpha$ confidence limits for σ^2. Likewise, their square roots are the $1-\alpha$ confidence limits for σ.

> *Example 7.3.*   The data of Example 7.1 can be assumed to come from a normal pop-
> ulation   (as will be demonstrated in Section 15.2). From this data, we have calculat-
> ed $s^2 = 320.27$,   and we now use it to find a 90% confidence interval for σ. We have
> $1-\alpha = .90$, so that $\alpha/2 = .05$. Since $n = 51$, the Chi-square variable has 50 degrees
> of freedom, and from Table III in the Appendix, corresponding to 50 degrees of
> freedom and .05 probabilities in the tails, we find $\chi^2(.95) = 34.76$ and $\chi^2(.05) = 67.50$.
> Therefore, with 90% confidence, we can assert that σ^2 falls between
> $(50)(320.27)/34.76 = 460.69$ and $(50)(320.27)/67.50 = 237.24$.   That   is,
> $237.24 \leqslant \sigma^2 \leqslant 460.69$. Hence, $15.4 \leqslant \sigma \leqslant 21.5$.

7.5. HYPOTHESIS TESTING

As in the case of the parameter p, the test of the hypothesis that specifies a value for
the parameter σ depends on the nature of the alternative hypothesis. In all cases, the
appropriate test statistic is the sample variance s^2 whose distribution is completely specified (for normal samples) once the value of σ^2 is given. In fact, when $\sigma^2 = \sigma_0^2$,

$$Y_0 = \frac{(n-1)s^2}{\sigma_0^2} \qquad (7.7)$$

has a Chi-square distribution with $n-1$ degrees of freedom. Since s^2 is an unbiased estimate of σ^2 , it is expected to be large when σ^2 is large and small when σ^2 is small. The
same is true of Y_0. We now consider using the statistic Y_0 in testing hypotheses about
σ at level α.

(i) This is the case that is mostly likely to be encountered in practice, when variability is suspected to be too high.

For testing $H_0 : \sigma^2 = \sigma_0^2$ against $H_R : \sigma^2 > \sigma_0^2$

or $H'_0 : \sigma^2 \leqslant \sigma_0^2$ against $H_R : \sigma^2 > \sigma_0^2$

the significant values are given by

$$Y_0 > \chi^2_{n-1} (\alpha), \tag{7.8}$$

where $\chi^2_{n-1} (\alpha)$ is the percentile of the Chi-square distribution with $n-1$ degrees of freedom that is exceeded with probability α.

(ii) For testing $H_0 : \sigma^2 = \sigma_0^2$ against $H_L : \sigma^2 < \sigma_0^2$

or $H'_0 : \sigma^2 \geqslant \sigma_0^2$ against $H_L : \sigma^2 < \sigma_0^2$

the significant values are given by

$$Y_0 < \chi^2_{n-1} (1-\alpha) \cdot \tag{7.9}$$

(iii) For testing $H_0 : \sigma^2 = \sigma_0^2$ against $H_T : \sigma^2 \neq \sigma_0^2$

the significant values are given by

$$Y_0 < \chi^2_{n-1} (1-\alpha/2)   \text{or}   Y_0 > \chi^2_{n-1} (\alpha/2). \tag{7.10}$$

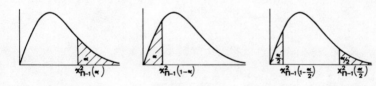

FIG. 7.2. Percentiles of a Chi-square distribution

Example 7.4.   With reference to the data in Example 7.1, suppose it is claimed that the calcium content in the Bekaa and South Lebanon is more variable than a specified standard deviation, say 15 mg/1. We state the hypothesis tested and alternative as $H_0 : \sigma \leqslant 15$ and $H_R : \sigma > 15$. Taking a significance level of 5%, we find $\chi^2_{50}(.05)$ in Table III in the Appendix to be 67.50. Using the calculated value of s^2 as in (7.7), we have $Y_0 = (50)(320.27)/225 = 71.17$ which is larger than $\chi^2_{50}(.05)$, and we therefore reject H_0 at the 5% level.

REFERENCES

Acra, A. (1975). *personal communication.* Department of Environmental Health, American University of Beirut, Beirut, Lebanon.

Pearson, E.S. and Hartley, H.O. (editors) (1966). *Biometrika Tables for Statisticians,* vol. I, 3rd ed., Cambridge University Press, Cambridge, England.

CHAPTER 8
The Mean of a
Numerical Variable

8.1. INTRODUCTION

The population mean μ is perhaps the most useful single summary measure of a population characteristic and the first to be investigated. As a measure of location, it can be very easily estimated and, as will be seen in later sections, the estimate has some attractive distributional properties which facilitate the application of statistical inference methods.

The population median M, which coincides with the mean in populations with symmetrical probability distributions, is sometimes a useful additional measure of location in populations where extreme values are known to exist in one of the tails so that symmetry cannot be assumed. In such populations the distribution is said to be *skewed*; it is positively skewed if the right tail contains unusually large values, and negatively skewed if the extreme values occur in the left tail. This is illustrated in Figure 8.1, which also shows the mean and the median of each distribution. In general, the sign of the difference μ−M is indicative of the skewness of the distribution, being positive for distributions that are positively skewed, zero for symmetrical distributions, and negative for distributions that are negatively skewed. Estimates of μ and M can thus be used for a rough check on the symmetry of a distribution.

A simple method of testing a hypothesis about the population median will be given in Section 8.5 b. The bulk of this chapter will be concerned with inference concerning the population mean.

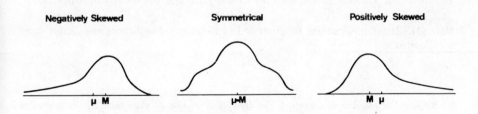

FIG. 8.1. The mean μ and the median M in three types of distributions

8.2. CALCULATION OF THE ESTIMATES

8.2 a. The Sample Mean

Given the observations $X_1, \ldots, X_n$ on a numerical variable, the most precise unbiased estimate of the population mean μ is the sample mean $\overline{X}$ defined as

$$\hat{\mu} = \overline{X} = \sum_{i=1}^{n} X_i/n. \tag{8.1}$$

The standard error of $\overline{X}$ is given by

$$\text{S.E.}(\overline{X}) = \sigma/\sqrt{n} \tag{8.2}$$

which depends on the population standard deviation σ. When σ is not known, as is often the case, this is replaced by the

$$\text{estimated S.E.}(\overline{X}) = s/\sqrt{n} \tag{8.3}$$

where s is the sample standard deviation. This quantity is part of the output of Program DESC2, as illustrated in Chapter 18.

Note (1). Equation (8.2) implies that the standard error of $\overline{X}$ is smaller when larger samples are taken from the same population. If σ is known, one can specify the maximum amount of standard error tolerated and find the necessary sample size to meet this condition by substituting the specified standard error in the left-hand side of (8.2) and solving the resulting equation for n. We shall return to this question in Section 8.4.

Note (2). If the sample is taken *without replacement* from a small population, the probabilities of the different possible values of X are changed with the drawing of each observation, and this change is reflected in the behavior of $\overline{X}$. As a result, the standard error of $\overline{X}$ is diminished by a factor which depends on the relative sizes of the population and sample, and becomes

$$\text{S.E.}(\overline{X}) = \frac{\sigma}{n}\sqrt{\frac{N-n}{N-1}}, \tag{8.4}$$

where N is the population size. The factor $(N-n)/(N-1)$ is called the *finite population correction* and is usually ignored when the sampling fraction, n/N, is less than 10 percent.

Note (3). If the observations are grouped in a frequency distribution, the sample mean is calculated as

$$\overline{X} = \sum_{i=1}^{k} f_i X_i/n, \tag{8.5}$$

where k is the number of classes, f_i the frequency in the ith class, and X_i the midpoint of the ith class interval. This quantity, as well as the sample median, are part of the output of Program DESC3 for grouped data, as illustrated in Chapter 18.

Example 8.1. We return to the data of Examples 7.1 and 7.2 (pp. 87, 88)
(i) Since $\Sigma X_i = 3209$, n = 51, $\overline{X} = 62.92$ by Formula (8.1).
(ii) Applying Formula (8.5) to the grouped data, we have from Example 7.2 that $\Sigma f_i X_i = 3255$, and therefore $\overline{X} = 63.82$, which is different from the earlier estimate because of the loss of some information in grouping.
(iii) In Example 7.1, σ was estimated as s = 17.9. Applying Formula (8.3), we obtain the estimate of the standard error of $\overline{X}$ as $17.9/\sqrt{51} = 2.51$. Combining (i) and (iii), we have the estimate 62.92 ± 2.51.

8.2 b. The Sample Median

Apart from being the logical estimate for the population median M, the sample median provides an alternative, and sometimes quicker, way of estimating the population mean. Also, since the sample median is not affected by extreme observations, it can be a more reliable estimate of μ than $\overline{X}$ when exceptionally large or exceptionally small values in the sample are suspected of being the result of observational error.

From a set of raw data, the median is obtained by first arranging the observations in ascending order, then locating the median as the middle observation (if their number is odd) or halfway between the two middle observations (if their number is even). Program DESC1 of Chapter 18 may be used to arrange the data.

If the observations are grouped in a frequency distribution, the class interval containing the sample median can be easily identified by an inspection of the cumulative frequencies, since the cumulative frequency for the previous class interval must be at most n/2 and the cumulative frequency for the interval itself must be at least n/2. Within this class interval whose lower boundary we denote by b, the median is usually located by interpolation : Let the difference between n/2 and the cumulative frequency up to the point b be denoted by d, the simple frequency in the class containing the median by f, and the width of this class interval by w. Then the median is taken as the point

$$b + (d)(w)/f. \tag{8.6}$$

These calculations will be illustrated in Example 8.2.

The standard error of the sample median, unlike that of the sample mean, depends on the type of distribution in the population. In samples from a normal population, the median, while also an unbiased estimate of μ, has a larger standard error than the mean. Roughly speaking, the standard error of the sample median is 1 to 1.25 times that of the sample mean in such populations, the exact ratio depending on the sample size and being larger for larger sample sizes (see, for instance, Kendall and Stuart, 1969).

Example 8.2. In this example, we again use the frequency distribution of calcium content in water samples of Example 7.2. Here, we calculate the median with reference to the histogram of the frequency distribution shown in Figure 8.2.

Since n = 51, the histogram represents 51 units of area, half of which (or 25.5) should fall to the left of the median. The area of the first four rectangles, being the cumulative frequency up to 60, is 22. Therefore d = 25.5 − 22 = 3.5. The frequency of the 5th interval is f = 13, so that the median is 60 + (3.5)(10)/13 = 62.69.

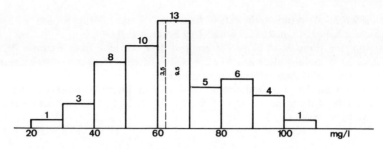

FIG. 8.2.   Locating the median in a frequency distribution

8.3.   SAMPLING DISTRIBUTION OF THE SAMPLE MEAN

As might be expected, the sampling distribution of the statistic $\overline{X}$ depends on the probability distribution of the variable X in the population. We have already seen, for example, that the mean of the sampling distribution is the same as the population mean μ and its standard deviation is equal to $\sigma/\sqrt{n}$, where σ is the population standard deviation. In addition, one expects the *shape* of the sampling distribution to be determined by the shape of the distribution of X. This is true in normal samples, where the sample mean $\overline{X}$ is also of the normal type, and in small samples from other distributions. Fortunately, however, if the sample is sufficiently large, the sampling distribution of $\overline{X}$ is little affected by the distribution of X, and one need not take the latter into account when using $\overline{X}$ in making inferences about μ.

In general, if X has *any* distribution with mean μ and standard deviation σ, and if $\overline{X}$ is the mean of a sample of size n where n is a large number, the sampling distribution of the standardized variable

$$\frac{\overline{X} - \mu}{\sigma/\sqrt{n}}$$

can be assumed to be that of the standard normal.

This very useful rule, which applies to both continuous and discrete variables, is due to an important theorem in statistical theory known as the *Central Limit Theorem.* Its validity will be demonstrated in a sampling experiment described in Example 8.3.

The only ambiguity in the above rule is the question of sample size, since it is not made clear what the number n must be for the sample to be considered "large". The fact is that, except in the case where X is itself a normal variable, the standard normal is only an approximation to the sampling distribution of the standardized $\overline{X}$, and while the approximation may be good with samples of size 10 from one population it may require samples of size 20 or more from another. By and large, the closer the distribution in the parent population is to the normal, the smaller the sample size needed for a good approximation. Also, whatever the distribution in the parent population may be, the approximation is better for larger samples. In the case of a normal X, the standard normal is the exact distribution of the standardized $\overline{X}$, however small the sample may be.

Example 8.3. In this example we describe the outcome of a sampling experiment in which samples have been taken from a non-normal population to study the variation in $\overline{X}$ from sample to sample and to check the suitability of the normal approximation. We took as our population 166 determinations of an index of sea-water intrusion (being the ratio of calcium to magnesium content) for water samples from certain regions in Lebanon (Acra, 1975). The population values were grouped in a frequency distribution whose frequency polygon is represented by the solid line in Figure 8.3. It is clear from this graph that the distribution of the index is far from normal.

Using a table of random digits, we took 100 samples of size 5 each from this population, sampling being done with replacement. For each sample, we calculated $\overline{X}$, and then grouped the $\overline{X}$ values in a frequency distribution whose frequency polygon is represented by the broken line in Figure 8.3. This process was repeated for samples of size 10, whose sample means were distributed as in the frequency polygon with the dotted line in Figure 8.3. Since a large number of $\overline{X}$ values was used for each of these frequency distributions, they can be considered as fairly good representations of the corresponding sampling distributions of the statistics.

Comparing the distributions of $\overline{X}$ with the distribution of X in the parent population, we see that
(i) in both cases, n = 5 and n = 10, the distribution of $\overline{X}$ is centered at the population mean μ, which was calculated from the population as 6.44;
(ii) the scatter of the values of $\overline{X}$ about μ is smaller in the case of the larger sample; and
(iii) although the original population distribution was highly skewed, the sampling distribution of $\overline{X}$ when n = 10 is reasonably close to the shape of the normal distribution.

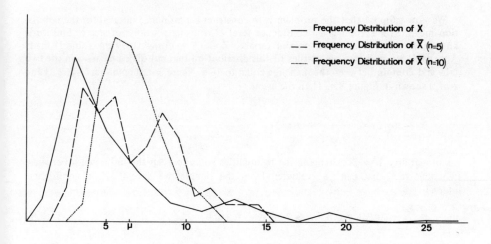

FIG. 8.3. Frequency distributions of X and $\overline{X}$ (Example 8.3)

One difficulty in using the sampling distribution of $\overline{X}$ in inference problems is the fact that the distribution depends on σ as well as on μ. We remark in passing that such a difficulty was not encountered in Chapter 7 in connection with the estimate of σ^2, for in that case the sampling distribution of the estimate depended only on σ^2. In the estimation of μ by $\overline{X}$, σ is a "nuisance parameter" whose value we need although we are interested only in the value of another parameter. There is no difficulty, of course, if σ is known. If σ is unknown, as is often the case, the difficulty is overcome by using s in the place of σ when standardizing $\overline{X}$. The resulting variable

$$T = \frac{\overline{X} - \mu}{s/\sqrt{n}} \tag{8.7}$$

is not a normal variable, however, even when the original distribution of X is normal. As shown by the following informal argument, this variable has a Student's t-distribution with n−1 degrees of freedom. To see this, consider the standard normal variable $Z = (\overline{X} - \mu)/(\sigma/\sqrt{n})$ and the variable $Y = (n-1)s^2/\sigma^2$ which has a Chi-square distribution with n−1 degrees of freedom. It is known that Z and Y are independent; therefore the ratio $Z/\sqrt{Y/(n-1)}$ has a t-distribution with n−1 degrees of freedom (see Section 4.4 f). But this is precisely the variable T defined in Equation (8.7)

As can be seen in figure 4.13, the density curve of the t-distribution is very well approximated by the normal curve when the parameter of T (the degrees of freedom) is not small. It is common practice to use the tables of the standard normal distribution instead of the t-tables when the degrees of freedom are 30 or more.

8.4. CONFIDENCE INTERVALS FOR μ

8.4 a.   When σ is known

We now suppose that the problem is to construct a confidence interval for the population mean, at a certain given confidence level $1-\alpha$, using a sample of size n. Since σ is known, we use the standard normal variable $Z = (\overline{X} - \mu)/(\sigma/\sqrt{n})$. From Table II in the Appendix, we find two percentiles of this distribution that cut off equal areas in the two tails and contain between them an area equal to $1-\alpha$. These are the numbers $-z(\alpha/2)$ and $z(\alpha/2)$ shown in Figure 8.4. Then the event

$$-z(\alpha/2) \leqslant \frac{\overline{X} - \mu}{\sigma/\sqrt{n}} \leqslant z(\alpha/2)$$

.has probability $1-\alpha$. Rearranging the inequalities so as to keep the unknown μ between two quantities that can be evaluated from the sample, we have the $1-\alpha$ confidence interval

$$\overline{X} - z(\alpha/2). \sigma/\sqrt{n} \leqslant \mu \leqslant \overline{X} + z(\alpha/2). \sigma/\sqrt{n}. \tag{8.8}$$

Confidence intervals for μ at 90, 95 or 99 percent confidence levels can also be obtained by means of Program MEAN1 of Chapter 18.

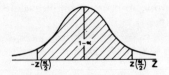

FIG. 8.4. Two percentiles of the standard normal distribution

Example 8.4. The standard deviation of the length of a certain species of crab is known to be $\sigma = 4.4$ mm. To estimate the mean length in the population, 16 specimens were selected at random from a catch and the length measured to the nearest tenth of a millimeter. The average length of the sample was found to be $\overline{X} = 25.5$ mm. For a confidence level of $1-\alpha = 90\%$, $z(\alpha/2) = 1.645$. Therefore a 90% confidence interval for μ is given by $25.5 \pm (1.645)(4.4)/\sqrt{16}$, or $(23.7, 27.3)$.

8.4 b. Precision and Sample size

By stating that the confidence interval for μ at level $1-\alpha$ is $\overline{X} \pm z(\alpha/2)$. $\sigma/\sqrt{n}$, we are essentially asserting that, at this level of confidence, $\overline{X}$ does not differ from μ by more than $z(\alpha/2)$. $\sigma/\sqrt{n}$. This quantity, then, is a measure of precision of the estimate and, since σ is known, the precision at any given level $1-\alpha$ can be improved by an increase in the sample size n. In particular, if it is required that, at level $1-\alpha$, the estimate $\overline{X}$ be within d units of the quantity estimated (where d is an arbitrary positive number), the sample to be taken must have size no less than n, where n is given by the condition $z(\alpha/2).\sigma/\sqrt{n} = d$, and therefore

$$n = (\frac{z(\alpha/2).\sigma}{d})^2 . \tag{8.9}$$

Example 8.5 In Example 8.4, if the mean length of this population of crab is to be estimated to within 1 mm of the true value at the 90% level of confidence, $d = 1$ and $z(\alpha/2) = 1.645$ and, since σ is known to be 4.4,

$$n = \left(\frac{(1.645)\,(4.4)}{1}\right)^2 = 52.39,$$

so that a sample of size 53 is required.

8.4 c. When σ is not known

When σ is not known, the confidence interval for μ is based on the variable $T = (\overline{X}-\mu)/(s/\sqrt{n})$ which has a Student's t-distribution with $n-1$ degrees of freedom. Let $t(\alpha/2)$ be that value of T which is exceeded with probability $\alpha/2$ as in Figure 8.5. Then the event.

$$-t\,(\alpha/2) \leqslant \frac{\overline{X}-\mu}{s/\sqrt{n}} \leqslant t\,(\alpha/2)$$

has probability $1-\alpha$ of occurring. As before, these inequalities can be rearranged to yield the $1-\alpha$ confidence interval for μ:

$$\overline{X}-t(\alpha/2).s/\sqrt{n} \leqslant \mu \leqslant \overline{X} +t(\alpha/2).s/\sqrt{n}. \tag{8.10}$$

For a given $1-\alpha$, and when n is known, $t(\alpha/2)$ can be obtained from Table IV in the Appendix.

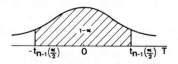

FIG. 8.5.   Two percentiles of the t-distribution with $n-1$ d.f.

If n is large $(n > 30)$, the percentiles of the t-distribution can be replaced by those of the standard normal distribution, and the $1-\alpha$ confidence interval for μ can be expressed as

$$\overline{X}-z(\alpha/2).s/\sqrt{n} \leqslant \mu \leqslant \overline{X} +z(\alpha/2) \tag{8.11}$$

Example 8.6.   In an experiment on the uptake of solutes by liver cells, Bikhazi (1978) found that six determinations of the radiation, measured in counts/min. after 20 minutes of immersion, were:

$$2726 \quad 2664 \quad 2587 \quad 2767 \quad 2875 \quad 2779.$$

The mean of these 6 observations is $\overline{X} = 2733$, and the standard deviation is $s = 99.56$. For $n-1 = 5$ degrees of freedom, and corresponding to a 90% level of confidence, which makes $\alpha/2 = .05$, we find that $t(\alpha/2) = 2.571$. Therefore the 90%confidence interval for the population mean of these observations is $2733 \pm (2.571)(99.56)/\sqrt{5}$ or $(2628.5, 2837.5)$.

8.5. HYPOTHESIS TESTING

8.5 a.   Testing hypotheses about μ

For testing hypotheses about the mean μ of a normal variable, we use the standardized statistic $\overline{X}$ whose distribution, as was seen in Section 8.3, can be considered as that of the standard normal — unless σ is unknown and n is 30 or less, in which case it is that of a t-variable with $n-1$ degrees of freedom.

In either case, since large values of $\overline{X}$ support hypotheses specifying large values of μ, and vice versa, it will be easy to see that the significant values of $\overline{X}$ in the following testing problems are as given in the corresponding rules. We again find it convenient to express these rules in terms of the standardized $\overline{X}$, and we use the notation $z(\alpha)$ to stand for the value of the standard normal variable exceeded with probability α and $t_{n-1}(\alpha)$ to stand for the corresponding value of a t-variable with $n-1$ degrees of freedom. We take α as the level of significance in each of these tests.

(i) $H_0 : \mu = \mu_0$ against $H_R : \mu > \mu_0$

or $H'_0 : \mu \leqslant \mu_0$ against $H_R : \mu > \mu_0$

The significant values of the test statistic are given by

$$\frac{\overline{X}-\mu_0}{\sigma /\sqrt{n}} > z(\alpha) \tag{8.12}$$

or, if σ is unknown, by

$$\frac{\overline{X}-\mu_0}{s /\sqrt{n}} > t_{n-1}(\alpha) \tag{8.13}$$

where $t_{n-1}(\alpha)$ is replaced by $z(\alpha)$ when $n > 30$. The significant values of the standardized statistics are shown in Figure 8.6.

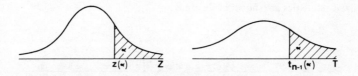

FIG. 8.6. Testing against a right-sided alternative at level α

(ii) $H_0 : \mu = \mu_0$ agianst $H_L : \mu < \mu_0$

or $H'_0 : \mu \geqslant \mu_0$ against $H_L : \mu < \mu_0$

The significant values are given by

$$\frac{\overline{X}-\mu_0}{\sigma /\sqrt{n}} < - z(\alpha) \tag{8.14}$$

or, if σ is unknown, by

$$\frac{\overline{X}-\mu_0}{s /\sqrt{n}} < - t_{n-1}(\alpha) \tag{8.15}$$

where $t_{n-1}(\alpha)$ is replaced by $z(\alpha)$ when $n > 30$. The significant values of the standardized statistics are shown in Figure 8.7.

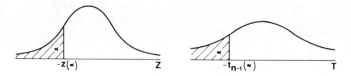

FIG. 8.7. Testing against a left-sided alternative at level α

(iii) $H_0 : \mu = \mu_0$ against $H_T : \mu \neq \mu_0$

The significant values are given by

$$\frac{|\overline{X}-\mu_0|}{\sigma/\sqrt{n}} > z(\alpha/2) \tag{8.16}$$

or, if σ is unknown, by

$$\frac{|\overline{X}-\mu_0|}{s/\sqrt{n}} > t_{n-1}(\alpha/2) , \tag{8.17}$$

where $t_{n-1}(\alpha/2)$ is replaced by $z(\alpha/2)$ when $n > 30$.   The significant values of the standardized   statistics are shown in Figure 8.8.

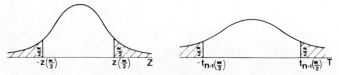

FIG. 8.8. Testing against a two-sided alternative at level α

Program MEAN2 of Chapter 18 may be used to calculate the t-statistics for the above tests.

Example 8.7.   The population of values of the "sea-water intrusion" index of Example 8.3 has a mean of 6.44 units, which was calculated from the data of that example. To check on whether a new locality has the same index on the average, we took 20 determinations of the index from samples taken from that locality and calculated :
$n = 20$, $\overline{X} = 6.03$, $s = 3.74$. We now use these results to test the hypothesis $H_0 : \mu = 6.44$ against $H_T : \mu \neq 6.44$ at the 5% level, where μ refers to the mean index of all possible samples from the new locality.

We first assume that σ is unknown, although in this case it can be found from the population data of Example 8.3. To use Formula (8.17), we look up t(.025) and find it equal to 2.093 for $n-1 = 19$. Since $|6.03\text{-}6.44|/(3.74/\sqrt{20}) = 0.49$ does not exceed 2.093. we accept H_0 at this level.

The P-value of the observed statistic is P($|T| \geqslant 0.49$), where T has 19 degrees of freedom. This probability is approximately 0.63.

If σ is actually calculated from the population values, the standardized statistic is no longer a t-variable, and the significant values of $\overline{X}$ are obtained by an application of Formula (8.16) instead of (8.17).

8.5 b. Testing hypotheses about the median

For any population with median M, suppose that we wish to test the hypothesis

$$H_0 : M = M_0 \quad \text{against } H_R : M > M_0 \,,$$

where M_0 is a specified number. To arrive at a suitable test statistic we observe that, when H_0 is true, the probability that any observation exceeds M_0 (which is the median) is $1/2$; on the other hand, when H_R is true, the probability that an observation exceeds M_0 (which is smaller than the median) is more than $1/2$ (see Figure 8.9). We therefore take as test statistic the number of observations, say R, that exceed M_0. Since R tends to

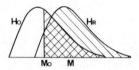

FIG. 8.9. $P(X > M_0)$ under H_0 and under H_R

be larger under H_R than under H_0, we reject the null hypothesis if R is too large. Now if H_0 is true, R is a binomial variable with parameters n and $p_0 = 1/2$ (Section 4.4 a) where n is the number of observations that differ from M_0, while if H_R is true it is a binomial variable with the same n but with a p larger than $1/2$. The testing problem is therefore identical with the problem in Section 6.5(i) and, if the normal approximation to the binomial can be used, the significant values of R are given by Formula (6.5) as

$$\frac{R - n/2 - 1/2}{\sqrt{n/4}} > z(\alpha),$$

that is, $\quad \dfrac{2R - n - 1}{\sqrt{n}} > z(\alpha).$

$$(8.18)$$

Since the normal approximation can be used whenever the smaller of np and $n(1-p)$ is at least 5, and the parameter p in this case is equal to $1/2$, we can use the normal approximation with samples in which n is at least 10. If n is smaller than 10, the significant values of R are found in the right tail of the binomial distribution with $p = 1/2$ by means of a table of the binomial probabilities or Program PROB2.

When the test is carried out against a left-sided alternative, the significant values of R are in the left tail of the distribution under M_0 and, if $n \geqslant 10$, the significant values are

$$\frac{2R - n + 1}{\sqrt{n}} < -z(\alpha).$$

$$(8.19)$$

Similarly, in testing H_0 against a two-sided alternative, and if $n \geq 10$, the significant values are

$$\frac{|2R-n|-1}{\sqrt{n}} > z(\alpha/2) \tag{8.20}$$

where α is the level of significance.

This is an easy test to apply. To calculate R, we look at each of the differences $X_i - M_0$ where X_i is the ith observation, and simply note whether each difference is positive, negative or zero. Then R is the number of positive differences, and n is the number of non-zero differences. Since the test is based on the sign of the differences, ignoring their magnitude, it is known as the *Sign Test*. Another use of the Sign Test will be described in Chapter 16.

Example 8.8. The median age of histologically confirmed cancer cases in Lebanon in the period August 1964 to July 1965 inclusive was calculated from a frequency distribution of these cases (Abou-Daoud, 1966) as 53.4. A sample of ages of such cases in 1978-79 was as follows: 49, 78, 56, 32, 39, 57, 66, 29, 54, 55. The question is: Is the median age M in 1978-79 the same as in the previous period or is it different? To test $H_0 : M = 53.4$ against $H_T : M \neq 53.4$ at the 5% level, we count the number of observations greater than 53.4 and find it to be $R = 6$. Applying (8.20), we have $(|12-10|-1)/\sqrt{10} = .32$, which is well below $z(.025) = 1.96$. Therefore the observed R is not significant, and the null hypothesis is accepted at the 5% level.

REFERENCES

Abou-Daoud, K.T. (1966). Morbidity from cancer in Lebanon. Cancer, *19*, 1293-1300.

Acra, A. (1975). *personal communication*. Department of Environmental Health, American University of Beirut, Lebanon.

Kendall, M.G. and Stuart, A. (1969). *The Advanced Theory of Statistics*, vol. I, 3rd ed., Charles Griffin and Co., London, England.

CHAPTER 9
The Difference
Between Two Means

9.1. INTRODUCTION

In comparing two samples, the investigator is usually seeking an answer to the question of whether or not they come from essentially the same population. The answer is seldom obvious for, even when the two samples do originate in the same population, they rarely give identical information, and one must decide whether the discrepancy may be simply attributed to chance variations or is due to intrinsic differences between the parent populations. Stated differently, the decision to be taken is between accepting the two sets of observations as observations on the same variable or as observations on two variables with different distributions.

For testing the equality of two distributions of a quantitative variable without any specific reference to their parameters, several "nonparametric tests" may be used, and some of these will be described in Chapter 16. In this chapter, we consider that aspect of the distributions which is most frequently of interest, namely their means. Comparing standard deviations of quantitative variables will be discussed in Chapter 11 and comparing the proportions of qualitative variables in Chapter 12.

Given two quantitative variables, suppose that we wish to investigate whether their population means are equal or, regardless of equality, to estimate the difference between the means. The methods that are used in these inference problems depend on the way in which the two samples are drawn from the two populations and whether they are "paired" or "independent".

Paired Samples, or what is often called "matched pairs", are those in which every observation from one population is matched with exactly one in the other, so that the observations come in pairs, and it is the differences in individual pairs that reflect differences between the population means.

Example 9.1. Edward *et al* (1977) studied lead poisoning in children of production workers in lead plants by matching families of workers with "control" families no member of which worked in a lead plant. Each of the matched pairs of families lived in the same neighborhood, had children in the same age group, houses of comparable ages, and had comparable levels of lead in painted surfaces. The effects of all these factors were thus eliminated or minimized in the comparison of the two groups.

Example 9.2. Another method of forming matched pairs is that of making the two observations on the same subject under two different conditions. Ruckebusch and Bueno (1976), in investigating the effects of feeding on the motility of the stomach and small intestine of a pig, measured the activity of these organs in each of 5 pigs both after 24 hours of fasting and following a certain pattern of feeding. By observing the same subject in the two situations, the effects of animal to animal variations are minimized.

Obviously, when the samples are paired, exactly the same number of observations is taken from each population.

Independent Samples. In such samples, n_1 observations are taken from the first population and n_2 observations from the second, where n_1 and n_2 may or may not be equal. Since there is no connection between an individual observation in one sample and any observation in the other, the recording of the data can be made in any order, as long as the two sets of observations are recorded separately. This method of drawing the samples is the one more commonly used, since it allows a lot of freedom in the choice of observations.

9.2. PAIRED SAMPLES

9.2 a. The Estimate and its Sampling Distribution

As we saw in Examples 9.1 and 9.2, a matched pair may be two observations on the same subject made before and after a certain treatment, or two observations made on two similar subjects one of which is "treated" and the other a "control". Wherever possible, once a pair of similar subjects is selected, they should be assigned the roles of "treated" and "control" at random, the randomization being repeated independently for each pair. This was impossible in Example 9.1, where the treatment was not experimentally administered, but such randomizations are always possible in a *clinical trial* in which the pairs of subjects are selected from a common pool of elements, and it is only when the treatment is administered to one member of each pair (at random) that the two samples are distinguishable. Matched pairs can also be taken as two observations on the same subject to which two treatments are administered on different occasions − provided, of course, that the first treatment in no way influences the observation on the second. In such an experiment, the order in which each subject receives the treatments should be made at random, say by drawing a random digit and assigning Treatment I first if the digit is odd or Treatment II first if the digit is even or zero.

In comparing two populations, it is immaterial which one of them is labelled as the first and which as the second. However, once the labels have been assigned, the order must be kept in mind when recording the observations and in making the subsequent calculations. Since the main interest in paired samples is in the differences, the n pairs of observations can be immediately summarized in the form of n differences, $D_1, \ldots, D_n$, where each D_i is the ith observation from Population I minus the corresponding observation from Population II. By considering the data as a sample of n differences, we are in effect replacing the two original populations by a single population, that of all possible

differences within pairs taken from populations I and II. Let $\mu(D)$ denote the mean of this population. Then $\mu(D)$ is the parameter that summarizes the difference between the means of populations I and II, and the problem of investigating that difference is reduced to the problem of investigating the value of an unknown population mean. This problem of a single population was dealt with in Chapter 8, and the results of that chapter can now be applied to the present problem. In particular, with a sample of n differences, $D_1, \ldots, D_n$, Formulas (8.1), (8.2) and (8.3) reduce to the following: $-$
As an estimate of $\mu(D)$, we use the sample mean of the differences

$$\bar{D} = \sum_{i=1}^{n} D_i/n, \tag{9.1}$$

which is an unbiased estimate of $\mu(D)$ with standard error

$$\text{S.E.}(\bar{D}) = \sigma(D)/\sqrt{n}, \tag{9.2}$$

where $\sigma(D)$ is the standard deviation in the population of differences. Since it is very unlikely that $\sigma(D)$ be known, we usually calculate the

$$\text{estimated S.E.}(\bar{D}) = s(D)/\sqrt{n}, \tag{9.3}$$

where $s(D)$, by analogy with Formula (7.2), is the square root of

$$s^2(D) = \frac{\sum\limits_{i=1}^{n} D_i^2 - (\sum\limits_{i=1}^{n} D_i)^2/n}{n-1}. \tag{9.4}$$

Moreover, as in Section 8.3, the approximate distribution of the standardized statistic

$$T = \frac{\bar{D} - \mu(D)}{s(D)/\sqrt{n}}$$

is a t-distribution with $n-1$ degrees of freedom or, for $n > 30$, the distribution of a standard normal variable.

9.2 b. Confidence Intervals and Tests for $\mu(D)$

By analogy with Formula (8.10), the confidence interval for $\mu(D)$ at level $1-\alpha$ is given by

$$\bar{D} - t_{n-1}(\alpha/2).s(D)/\sqrt{n} \leqslant \mu(D) \leqslant \bar{D} + t_{n-1}(\alpha/2).s(D)/\sqrt{n}, \tag{9.5}$$

where $t_{n-1}(\alpha/2)$ is the $100(1-\alpha/2)$ percentile of the t-distribution with $n-1$ degrees of freedom, as in Figure 8.5.

By analogy with Section 8.5, the test statistic for any hypothesis concerning the value of $\mu(D)$ is the estimate $\bar{D}$. As before, the test will be one-tailed or two-tailed depending on whether the alternative is one-sided or two-sided. The significant values of the test statistic in each case are given by Formulas (8.13), (8.15) and (8.17) in which $\overline{D}$ should be substituted for $\overline{X}$, $\mu(D)$ for μ, and s(D) for s. (see pages 101, 102).

Note We have based the above methods on the t-distribution because we considered it highly unlikely that the standard deviation of this hypothetical population of differences was known. If $\sigma(D)$ can be assumed to be known (from previous investigations on similar variables, perhaps), then the known value is used instead of the estimated value s(D), and the standard normal distribution is used instead of the t-distribution.

Example 9.3 In a series of experiments on the temporal and masseter muscles of the cat, Tamari *et al* (1973) found significant differences in several of the muscle characteristics. To illustrate the inference methods of this section, we have selected their data on tetanus frequency of the muscles of 9 cats before and after the injection of a certain dose of tubocurarine. This data is reproduced in Table 9.1.

Table 9.1. Comparison of tetanus frequency (in Hz)
in the temporal (T) and masseter (M) muscles
before and after injection of tubocurarine

Cat	T Before	M Before	T After	M After
1	32	38	30	34
2	24	34	28	30
3	28	34	20	30
4	30	37	30	37
5	30	34	20	28
6	28	28	29	29
7	24	28	24	28
8	24	28	24	28
9	20	42	18	38

Source : Tamari *et al* (1973)

We first use the tetanus frequency before injection to estimate the mean difference in that frequency between the temporal and masseter muscles by a 95% confidence interval. The nine differences ("masseter" minus "temporal") are :

6   10   6   7   4   0   4   4   22.

Using these figures, we calculate $\overline{D} = 7$, $s(D) = 6.24$. For $1-\alpha = .95$, $\alpha/2 = .025$ and, from the t-tables at 8 degrees of freedom, we find $t_8(.025) = 2.306$. Substituting in Formula (9.5), we arrive at the 95% confidence interval (2.20, 11.80). We observe that, since this interval does not contain the zero point, a 5% level two-tailed test of the hypothesis that $\mu(D) = 0$ would be rejected.

We next consider the 9 pairs of observations on the masseter muscle before and after injection to test the null hypothesis that the injection has no effect on the tetanus frequency of the muscle, against a two-sided alternative, at the 5% level. The null hypothesis is $H_0: \mu(D) = 0$, and the alternative hypothesis is $H_T: \mu(D) \neq 0$. In this case, the nine differences ("Before" minus "After") are:

$$4 \quad 4 \quad 4 \quad 0 \quad 6 \quad -1 \quad 0 \quad 0 \quad 4.$$

Using these figures, we calculate $\overline{D} = 2.33$ and $s(D) = 2.55$. Since $\alpha/2 = .025$ and $n = 9$, we again have $t_8 (.025) = 2.306$. Therefore, by a formula analogous to (8.17), we would reject H_0 if $\overline{D}/(2.55/3) > 2.306$. Since $\overline{D}/(2.55/3) = 2.74$, we reject the null hypothesis and conclude, at this significance level, that the injection does have an effect on the tetanus frequency of the masseter muscle.

To calculate the P-value of the observed mean difference, we look in the t-tables at 8 degrees of freedom for the probability of the standardized $\overline{D}$ being 2.74 or a more extreme value in either of the two tails. This is a little over 2% but cannot be evaluated more accurately because of the limited number of percentiles provided by our table of the t-distribution. It is interesting to note that, since the P-value of our statistic is more than 2%, if we had decided to perform the test of H_0 against H_T at the 2% instead of the 5% level, the null hypothesis would have been accepted.

9.3. INDEPENDENT SAMPLES

9.3 a. The Estimate and Its Sampling Distribution

Consider two populations with means μ_1 and μ_2 and variances σ_1^2 and σ_2^2, and suppose that a set of n_1 observations are taken on the first variable and, quite independently, another set of n_2 observations are taken on the second. The object is to use these $n_1 + n_2$ observations to investigate the difference, if any, between μ_1 and μ_2.

The parameter of interest, then, is $\theta = \mu_1 - \mu_2$, and the obvious estimate of this parameter is $\overline{X}_1 - \overline{X}_2$, or the corresponding difference between the sample means. Being the difference of two unbiased estimates of the two means, $\overline{X}_1 - \overline{X}_2$ is an unbiased estimate of $\mu_1 - \mu_2$. Its standard error is

$$\text{S.E.}(\overline{X}_1 - \overline{X}_2) = \sqrt{\frac{\sigma_1^2}{n_1} + \frac{\sigma_2^2}{n_2}} \tag{9.6}$$

This formula derives from the fact that if two variables are independent, the variance of their difference is the sum of their variances, and the fact that each of the sample means has a variance whose square root is given by Formula (8.2).

Formula (9.6) is of no practical use in calculating the standard error of the estimate unless σ_1 and σ_2 are known. If they are, and if n_1 and n_2 are not very small, the standardized statistic

$$Z = \frac{(\overline{X}_1 - \overline{X}_2) - (\mu_1 - \mu_2)}{\sqrt{\dfrac{\sigma_1^2}{n_1} + \dfrac{\sigma_2^2}{n_2}}} \tag{9.7}$$

has approximately a standard normal distribution.

If the population standard deviations are not known, the situation is a little more complicated than in the single-sample case where the unknown standard deviation was replaced by its estimate and the resulting standardized statistic had a well-defined distribution. Here, we have two cases: (i) the case where σ_1 and σ_2, although unknown, are assumed or known to be equal, and (ii) the case where they cannot be assumed equal and therefore constitute two nuisance parameters.

(i) **The case where** $\sigma_1 = \sigma_2$. Let their common value be denoted by σ, so that Formula (9.6) can be written as

$$\text{S.E.}(\overline{X}_1 - \overline{X}_2) = \sigma \sqrt{\frac{1}{n_1} + \frac{1}{n_2}} \; .$$

The variance σ^2 has an unbiased estimate, called the "pooled estimate" of variance (because the resources of both samples are pooled together in this estimate), and defined by

$$s_p^2 = \frac{(n_1 - 1)s_1^2 + (n_2 - 1)s_2^2}{n_1 + n_2 - 2} \tag{9.8}$$

where s_1^2 and s_2^2 are the two sample variances, each calculated as in Formula (7.2). Using the square root of s_p^2 as the estimate of the unknown σ, we have the standardized statistic

$$T = \frac{(\overline{X}_1 - \overline{X}_2) - (\mu_1 - \mu_2)}{s_p \sqrt{\dfrac{1}{n_1} + \dfrac{1}{n_2}}} \tag{9.9}$$

which has a t-distribution with $n_1 + n_2 - 2$ degrees of freedom. We observe that the degrees of freedom of the t-variable are those of s_p^2 and represent the total number of unrestricted variables involved in defining it.

(ii) **The case where** $\sigma_1 \neq \sigma_2$ **and both are unknown.** In this case, the only possibility open to us is to replace each unknown standard deviation by its estimate from the corresponding sample, so that the standardized form of the estimate becomes

$$U = \frac{(\overline{X}_1 - \overline{X}_2) - (\mu_1 - \mu_2)}{\sqrt{\dfrac{s_1^2}{n_1} + \dfrac{s_2^2}{n_2}}} \cdot \qquad (9.10)$$

Even when the parent populations are normal, this variable has neither the standard normal nor the t-distribution. For certain probability levels in the normal case, percentiles of this variable can be obtained from special tables (see Pearson and Hartley, 1966, Table 11).

Note (1). The variances of two populations can be assumed equal when the nature of the variable is such that any difference between the populations is essentially a difference between their means, or if previous investigations on the same variable suggest the equality of the variances.

Note (2). A test of the hypothesis that the variances of two normal populations are equal will be given in Section 11.2. The test depends only on the sample variances and can be easily carried out. However, if the parent populations are far from normal, conclusions based on this test may be open to question.

Note (3). In the one-sample problem, we found that the probabilities of a t-variable could be well approximated by those of the standard normal variable if the sample size exceeded 30. In terms of the parameter of the t-variable, the condition is that the degrees of freedom should be at least 30. Therefore, in the two-sample problem of this section, the condition for replacing a t-percentile by the corresponding z-percentile becomes: $n_1 + n_2 - 1 \geqslant 30$.

9.3 b. Confidence Intervals and Tests for $\mu_1 - \mu_2$

With the exception of Case (ii), in which the standard deviations of the two populations were unknown and unequal, and which will be treated separately at the end of this section, the formulas giving confidence intervals and rules for testing hypotheses about the parameter $\theta = \mu_1 - \mu_2$ are identical in form to the corresponding formulas for the single parameter μ. In both cases, the rules are based on a standardized variable which has the form

$$\frac{\text{(Estimate)} - \text{(Parameter)}}{\text{S.E.(Estimate)}}$$

and has a standard normal distribution if S.E (Estimate) is known. If the unknown σ in this standard error is replaced by an estimate, s, the resulting standardized variable has the t-distribution with as many degrees of freedom as in the denominator of s^2.

Starting with the formulas of Sections 8.4 and 8.5, we replace μ by $\mu_1 - \mu_2$, $\overline{X}$ by $\overline{X}_1 - \overline{X}_2$, S.E.($\overline{X}$) by S.E.($\overline{X}_1 - \overline{X}_2$), and the n−1 degrees of freedom by $n_1 + n_2 - 2$. The resulting rules for confidence intervals, at level $1-\alpha$, and for the tests at significance level α, are listed below. As usual, $z(\alpha)$ denotes the $100(1-\alpha)$ percentile of the standard normal distribution, $t_{n_1 + n_2 - 2}(\alpha)$ (or simply $t(\alpha)$) denotes the corresponding percentile of the t-distribution with $n_1 + n_2 - 2$ degrees of freedom, and the t percentile can be replaced by the z percentile if $n_1 + n_2 - 2 \geqslant 30$. These constants are shown in Figure 9.1.

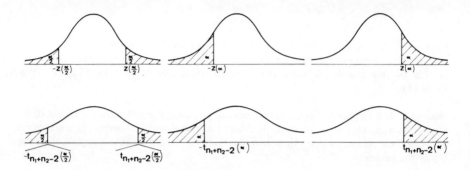

FIG. 9.1.   Percentiles of the standard normal distribution and
the t-distribution with $n_1 + n_2 - 2$ d.f.

Confidence intervals: σ_1 and σ_2 known. The confidence limits are given by

$$(\bar{X}_1 - \bar{X}_2) \pm z(\alpha/2) \sqrt{\frac{\sigma_1^2}{n_1} + \frac{\sigma_2^2}{n_2}} \quad . \tag{9.11}$$

Confidence intervals: $\sigma_1 = \sigma_2$, unknown. The confidence limits are given by

$$(\bar{X}_1 - \bar{X}_2) \pm t(\alpha/2).s_p \sqrt{\frac{1}{n_1} + \frac{1}{n_2}} \tag{9.12}$$

where s_p is defined in Formula (9.8).

Tests of hypotheses: σ_1 and σ_2 known. The test statistic, standardized when $\theta = \theta_0$, is

$$Z_0 = \frac{\bar{X}_1 - \bar{X}_2 - \theta_0}{\sqrt{\frac{\sigma_1^2}{n_1} + \frac{\sigma_2^2}{n_2}}} \quad . \tag{9.13}$$

(i)   For testing $H_0 : \mu_1 - \mu_2 \leqslant \theta_0$ against $H_R : \mu_1 - \mu_2 > \theta_0$, the significant values are given by
$$Z_0 > z(\alpha). \tag{9.14}$$

(ii)   For testing $H_0 : \mu_1 - \mu_2 \geqslant \theta_0$ against $H_L : \mu_1 - \mu_2 < \theta_0$, the significant values are given by

$$Z_0 < -z(\alpha). \tag{9.15}$$

(iii)   For testing $H_0 : \mu_1 - \mu_2 = \theta_0$ against $H_T : \mu_1 - \mu_2 \neq \theta_0$, the significant values are given by

$$|Z_0| > z(\alpha/2) \tag{9.16}$$

Tests of hypotheses: $\sigma_1 = \sigma_2$, unknown. The test statistic, standardized when $\theta = \theta_0$, is

$$T_0 = \frac{\overline{X}_1 - \overline{X}_2 - \theta_0}{s_p \sqrt{\dfrac{1}{n_1} + \dfrac{1}{n_2}}}, \tag{9.17}$$

where s_p is defined in (9.8). By analogy with (9.14), (9.15) and (9.16), the significant values are given by:
For testing problem (i), $T_0 > t(\alpha)$. \hfill (9.18)

For testing problem (ii), $T_0 < - t(\alpha)$. \hfill (9.19)

For testing problem (iii), $|T_0| > t(\alpha/2)$. \hfill (9.20)

The corresponding program in Chapter 18 is Program MEAN3.

Example 9.4   In a study of factors affecting ischaemic heart disease (Logan *et al*, 1978), several physical characteristics of two groups of 40-year old men from Edinburgh and Stockholm were compared. We use only the data on their heights to illustrate the construction of confidence intervals from independent samples. The data relevant to our exercise is summarized in Table 9.2.

Table 9.2.   Mean heights (cm) of men in two independent samples

	Edinburgh	Stockholm
n	107	87
$\overline{X}$	173	179
s	6.0	7.0

Source : Logan *et al* (1978)

We assume that $\sigma_1 = \sigma_2$, which is suggested both by the nature of the variable and the fact that s_1 and s_2 are very close in value. By formula (9.8), we find that

$$s_p^2 = \frac{(106)(36) + (86)(49)}{192} \qquad \text{so that } s_p = 6.47.$$

For a confidence level of 90%, we have $\alpha/2 = .05$ and, since the degrees of freedom are 192, we use the standard normal tables and find $z(.05) = 1.645$. The interval is therefore, by (9.12), $-6 \pm (1.645)(6.47)(.1444)$, or $(-7.54, -4.46)$, which is the 90% confidence interval for the parameter: "Edinburgh population mean" minus "Stockholm population mean".

Example 9.5. In a survey of normal and pathological immunoglobulins in Lebanese and other Middle-Eastern populations, Alami (1978) determined immunoglobulin levels from a large number of blood samples representing both sexes and several different age groups. His data on IgD levels (in mg/100ml) for a sample of 13-years olds was as follows:

Male :	12.0	0.0	9.3	8.1	5.8	6.8	3.6	9.5	8.6	7.3
Female :	5.8	0.0	7.0	0.0	7.5	2.6	5.5	7.2	7.3	3.3

We use this data to test the hypothesis that there is no difference between the sexes in the mean level of IgD. We take 5% as our significance level and, in the absence of any stated one-sided alternative, we test against the two-sided alternatives that the mean levels are different. Again, let $\sigma_1 = \sigma_2$. We have the calculated quantities:

$$\overline{X}_1 = 7.10 \qquad\qquad \overline{X}_2 = 4.62$$

$$s_1^2 = 11.3711 \qquad\qquad s_2^2 = 8.7196$$

$$n_1 = 10 \qquad\qquad n_2 = 10$$

$$s_p = 3.17$$

Since $\theta_0 = 0$ calculate T_0 using (9.17) as

$$T_0 = \frac{(7.10 - 4.62)}{3.17\sqrt{0.2}} = 1.75 .$$

From the tables, $t_{18}(.025) = 2.101$. Applying (9.20), we see that $(\overline{X}_1 - \overline{X}_2)$ is not significant at the 5% level, since $T_0 < 2.101$. The P-value of the observed statistic is $P(|T_0| > 1.75) = 2P(T > 1.75) \cong .10$ from tables of the t-distribution with 18 degrees of freedom.

We now return to Case (ii) of Section 9.3 a and the difficulty of having two unknown variances. Several approximate solutions for the problems of confidence intervals and hypothesis testing in this case have been proposed. Perhaps the simplest to apply is the method that considers the variable U, which was defined in Formula (9.10), as approximately a t-variable with f degrees of freedom (Welch, 1949), where f is given by

$$f = \frac{(s_1^2/n_1 + s_2^2/n_2)^2}{(s_1^2/n_1)^2/(n_1-1) + (s_2^2/n_2)^2/(n_2-1)} \qquad\qquad (9.21)$$

If f is a fraction, the closest integer is taken as degrees of freedom. All the inference methods based on the t-distribution, namely those given in Formulas (9.12) and (9.17) to (9.20), can now be used if, instead of $n_1 + n_2 - 2$, the degrees of freedom are taken as f and if

$$s_p \sqrt{\frac{1}{n_1} + \frac{1}{n_2}} \quad \text{is replaced by} \quad \sqrt{\frac{s_1^2}{n_1} + \frac{s_2^2}{n_2}}. \qquad (9.22)$$

The corresponding program in Chapter 18 is Program MEAN4.

Example 9.6. In one of his experiments on the net conversion of Progesterone in rat liver, Salti (1970) obtained the following determinations of net conversion in rats 3-4 weeks old:

Males :	16.1	16.8	13.5	13.0	14.3	11.6	12.8
	17.5	12.8	8.9	16.0	16.8	16.7	15.2
Females :	14.6	11.1	7.0	10.4	15.8	14.6	9.4
	9.8	5.1	5.5	6.4	7.1		

To test $H_0: \mu_1 - \mu_2 = 0$ against $H_R: \mu_1 - \mu_2 > 0$, at the 1% level, we make the following calculations:

$$n_1 = 14, \ \bar{X}_1 = 14.4, \ s_1^2 = 6.04, \ s_1^2/n_1 = .4313,$$

$$n_2 = 12, \ \bar{X}_2 = 9.7, \ s_2^2 = 13.77, \ s_2^2/n_2 = 1.1478,$$

f = 18.60. Interpolating between 18 and 19 degrees of freedom, we get t(.01) = 2.545.

From (9.17) and (9.22), $T_0 = \dfrac{4.7 - 0}{\sqrt{.4313 + 1.1478}} = 3.74.$

According to (9.18), this is significant, and we reject the hypothesis of equality of mean net conversion.

REFERENCES

Alami, S.Y. (1978). *personal communication.* Department of Clinical Pathology, American University of Beirut, Beirut, Lebanon.

Baker E.L., Fallan, D.S., Taylor, T.A., Frank, M., Peterson, W., Lovejoy, G., Cox, D., Houseworth, J., and Landrigan, P. (1977). Lead poisoning in children of lead workers. New Engl. J. Med. *296*, 260-261.

Logan, R.L., Riemersma, R.A., Thomson, M., Oliver, M.F., Olsson, A.G., Walldius, G., Rössner, S., Kaijser, L., Callmer, E., Carlson, L.A., Lockerbie, L. and Lutz, W. (1978). Risk functions for ischaemic heart-disease in normal men aged 40. Lancet, 6 May 1978, 949-954.

Pearson, E.S. and Hartley, H.O. (editors) (1966). *Biometrika Tables for Statisticians,* vol. I, 3rd ed., Cambridge University Press, Cambridge, England.

Ruckebusch, Y. and Bueno, L. (1976). The effect of feeding on the motility of the stomach and small intestine in the pig. Br. J. Nutr. *35,* 397-405.

Salti, I.S. (1970). 16 α–hydroxylation of Progesterone by rat liver, Ph.D. thesis, University of Toronto.

Tamari, J.W., Tomey, G.F., Ibrahim. M.Z.M., Baraka, A., Jabbur, S., and Bahuth, N. (1973). Correlative study of the physiologic characteristics of the temporal and masseter muscles of the cat. J. dent. res. *52,* 538-543.

Welch, B. (1949). Further note on Mrs. Aspin's tables and on certain approximations to the tabled function. Biometrika, *36,* 293-296.

CHAPTER 10
Comparing Several Means

10.1. INTRODUCTION

When the means of more than two quantitative populations are to be compared, the methods of the previous chapter are not sufficient, although they can still be used to make comparisons between any two of the populations at a time. Situations involving several populations are common. The populations may be outcomes of different "treatments", possibly including a control, in a planned experiment, or they may be values of a variable resulting from conditions that are recognized as different but are beyond the investigator's control. In all such cases, the main problem is usually to find an answer to the following question: Given a sample from each of the populations, are the observed discrepancies among the sample means simply due to chance fluctuations, or are they due to intrinsic differences among the populations? It should be possible to find an answer to this question if one could somehow separate the effects of purely random variations from those caused by existing differences among population means. This is essentially what is accomplished by a technique called the *analysis of variance*, which will be used in this chapter.

Analysis of variance techniques are applicable to a wide variety of problems in which several sources of variation can be identified and classified. For each problem, the observations are taken in accordance with a properly designed plan, and the more sources of variation the investigator recognizes the more complex is the design of his "experiment". In the problem of comparing several means, we recognize two possible sources of variation: variation from population to population, and random variation within the populations. The observations are taken independently from each population (like the two-population independent sample case) and listed in what is known as a one-way (or single) classification. Such a plan for collecting the observations is called a *completely randomized design* because the choice of the random samples from the different populations is completely free. This distinguishes it from other designs in which (like the case of paired samples) an observation from one of the populations must be linked with exactly one from each of the other populations, to form a randomized "block". Randomized blocks or any of the other more complex designs are outside the scope of this book.

Having obtained the set of independent samples, and before embarking on the analysis of variance computations, the investigator will find it useful to examine the data by making a graphical representation of some summary statistics. The most commonly used summary consists of the means and standard deviations of the samples. The means are plotted on a separate vertical axis for each sample, then a line segment representing one standard deviation above and below the mean is drawn through it, as shown in Figure 10.1. Instead of plotting the points $\bar{X} \pm s$ for each sample, one can plot the smallest and largest X as well as $\bar{X}$ along the same vertical axis, so that the line segment joining them represents the sample range. This is a quicker method, since it avoids the calculation of the standard deviation of each sample. But unless the sample sizes are all equal, this representation may be misleading, since the range reflects a different multiple of the standard deviation in samples of different sizes, as can be seen from Table 7.1, page 87 .

Example 10.1.   The data in this example is taken from a larger set of data collected by Feisal *et al* (1961) in an investigation of the effect of chlorothiazide on responses to norepinephrine. We take as our populations the response to four doses of norepinephrine, 0, .075, .150, and .300 μg/lb/min., after 7 days of chlorothiazide treatment, where the response X is the mean blood pressure of normal human subjects in mm of Hg. Each sample consists of five observations. Since the sample sizes are all equal, we may use the sample range as a measure of sample variability in this preliminary investigation. The relevant summaries of the data are:

Dose	.000	.075	.150	.300
$\bar{X}$	86.0	94.6	104.8	110.8
Sample range	10	13	19	17

These are plotted on four different vertical axes in Figure 10.1. Although we are here interested only in the four populations as four different doses of norepinephrine (regardless of their relative magnitudes), the doses are marked to scale on the horizontal axis since such a marking requires no additional effort. Populations are not always defined in terms of a numerical quantity the way they are in this example, and their placing along the horizontal axis is in general quite arbitrary.

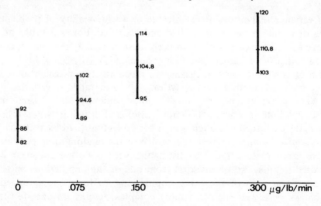

FIG. 10.1. The means and ranges of four samples (Example 10.1)

No formal inferences can be made from this graphical summary, but it does bring out some interesting features of the data. We notice, for instance, that the mean seems to increase with an increase in the dosage. This suggests a possible functional relationship between blood pressure and dosage, and a simple type of relationship (linear regression) can be investigated by the methods of Chapter 14. Moreover, the range (and therefore the standard deviation) is generally larger with the larger means. This may be purely a chance phenomenon, but it may also be a characteristic of the populations, in which case a transformation of the observations would be necessary before the analysis of variance is carried out. This matter will be discussed in Section 10.5 of this chapter.

10.2. THE MODEL

Consider k populations of the same variable X. The populations are variously referred to as "groups", "classes" or "treatments" by different authors, but whatever they are called they represent k distributions of X which may or may not be identical. Suppose that a sample of size n_i is taken from the ith population (where i is any of the numbers $1, \ldots, k$) and denote the jth observation in this sample by X_{ij}. The k samples then consist of the observations

$$X_{11}, X_{12}, \ldots, X_{1n_1}$$
$$X_{21}, X_{22}, \ldots, X_{2n_2}$$
$$. \ .$$
$$. \ .$$
$$X_{k1}, X_{k2}, \ldots \ldots, X_{kn_k},$$

whose total count is $n_1 + n_2 + \ldots + n_k = n$.

The analysis of variance methods that we use in this chapter are based on the assumption that, in each of the populations,

(i) X has a normal distribution;

(ii) X has an unknown mean, which we denote by μ_i for the ith population;

(iii) X has the same unknown variance in all the populations. As usual, we denote this variance by σ^2.

The main problem is to test the null hypothesis

$$H_0 : \mu_1 = \mu_2 = \ldots = \mu_k,$$

which implies that the populations are identical, against the very general alternative

$$H_A : \text{Not all the } \mu_i \text{ are equal.}$$

We notice that H_A covers a very wide range of situations, from the case where all but one of the population means are equal to the case where they are all different. Therefore, with such an alternative, if the samples lead us to reject H_0, we are left with a lot of unsettled questions about the means of the k populations. This problem is dealt with in Section 10.4.

10.3. TESTING THE HYPOTHESIS OF EQUAL MEANS

The analysis of variance test of H_0 consists of comparing two estimates of σ^2, an estimate based on variations from sample to sample and one based on variations within the samples, and rejecting the null hypothesis if the first estimate is so much larger than the second that the samples cannot be assumed to come from the same population. The calculations leading to the two estimates are carried out as described below:

$$\text{Let } T_i = \sum_{j=1}^{n_i} X_{ij} \quad \text{and} \quad T = \sum_{i=1}^{k} T_i,$$

so that T_i is the sum of all the observations in the ith sample, and T is the sum of all the observations in all the samples.

1) Calculate T^2/n. This quantity is sometimes called "the correction for the mean".

2) Calculate the sum of squares of all the individual observations, $\sum\sum X_{ij}^2$, and use it to calculate what is called the *total sum of squares.*

$$\text{SS(total)} = \sum_i \sum_j X_{ij}^2 - T^2/n.$$

This sum of squares involves all n variables with one restriction on them (their sum is T) and therefore has $n-1$ degrees of freedom.

3) Calculate the *sum of squares between samples,*

$$\text{SS(between)} = \sum_i T_i^2/n_i - T^2/n.$$

This sum of squares involves the k sample totals with one restriction on them (their sum is T) and thus has $k-1$ degrees of freedom.

4) Enter the results of steps 2 and 3 in an analysis of variance table, a model for which is shown in Table 10.1.

Table 10.1.   Analysis of variance for single classification

Source of Variation	Sum of Squares SS	Degrees of Freedom	Mean Square MS
Between samples	$\sum_{i=1}^{k} T_i^2/n_i - T^2/n$	$k-1$	
Within samples			
Total	$\sum_{i=1}^{k} \sum_{j=1}^{n_i} X_{ij}^2 - T^2/n$	$n-1$	

5) Calculate the difference: SS(total) $-$ SS(between) and enter the results in the table as the *sum of squares within samples,* SS(within). Although it is not obvious from the calculations, this difference is identical with the pooled sum of squared deviations for all k samples, that is, the quantity

$$\sum_{i=1}^{k} \sum_{j=1}^{n_i} (X_{ij} - \overline{X}_i)^2 ,$$

where $\overline{X}_i$ is the mean of the ith sample. Its degrees of freedom are also obtained by subtracting $k-1$ from $n-1$.

6) Divide SS(between) by its degrees of freedom to obtain the mean square, MS(Between), and enter the result in the table. This is the first estimate of σ^2. If H_0 is true, this estimate is unbiased, but it tends to be too large if H_0 is not true, that is, if the differences among sample means exceed the amount expected in random samples from the same population.

7) Divide SS(within) by its degrees of freedom to obtain the mean square, MS (within), which is an unbiased estimate of σ^2 no matter how alike or different the μ_i may be.

In view of the nature of these two estimates, as described in steps 6 and 7, a suitable test statistic for the null hypothesis is the ratio

$$R = MS(between) / MS(within)$$

which should be close to 1 if the hypothesis is true and larger if it is not true. This implies that the significant values of the test statistic are in the right tail of its distribution under H_0. Now this distribution is that of an F variable (see Section 4.4) with $k-1$ and $n-k$ degrees of freedom. This follows from the normality of the parent populations which makes each of the statistics SS(between) and SS(within), when divided by σ^2, a Chi-square variable with the corresponding degrees of freedom. These two statistics can also be shown to be independent, and therefore the ratio of the mean squares is the F variable mentioned above. The F distribution is sometimes referred to as the distribution of the *variance ratio*. The variance ratio R can also be obtained by means of Program MEAN5 of Chapter 18.

To test H_0 at significance level α, we compare the calculated value of R from the sample with its significant values

$$R > F_{k-1, n-k} (\alpha),$$

where $F_{k-1, n-k} (\alpha)$ is the percentile in the right tail of the F distribution with $k-1$ and $n-k$ degrees of freedom, as shown in Figure 10.2.

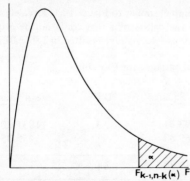

FIG. 10.2. The 100 $(1-\alpha)$ th percentile of the F−distribution with $(k-1, n-k)$ d.f.

Note (1). The estimate of variance in the denominator of the F ratio, namely MS(within), can be written as $\Sigma\Sigma(X_{ij}-\bar{X}_i)^2 / (n-k)$, which shows it to be the pooled estimate of variance from the k samples and analogous to the estimate of the common variance that was defined for two independent samples. In fact, if we take $k = 2$ in this formula, it reduces to Formula (9.8) of the previous chapter.

Note (2). Although the test based on the analysis of variance was introduced for more than two populations, there is nothing in the calculations that prevents k from being as small as 2. If $k = 2$, how does this test compare with the t-test for equality of means in independent samples that was given in Chapter 9? We have already seen that MS(within) $= s_p^2$ as defined in Formula (9.8). The numerator mean square MS(between), can be written in terms of $\bar{X}_1$ and $\bar{X}_2$ instead of T_1 and T_2 and simplifies to the form

$$\frac{(\bar{X}_1 - \bar{X}_2)^2}{\dfrac{1}{n_1} + \dfrac{1}{n_2}}\;.$$

Dividing this statistic by s_p^2, we get the square of the t-variable of (9.9) with $\mu_1 - \mu_2$ replaced by 0. Therefore values of F which are in the right tail of the F-distribution correspond to values of T which are in the two tails of the t-distribution, and the F-test when applied to 2 samples is equivalent to the two-tailed t-test of the hypothesis that $\mu_1 - \mu_2 = 0$.

Example 10.2. From the survey referred to in Example 9.5 (p.114), we have extracted the following random sample of observations on children under 10 years of age, each observation being the IgA immunoglobulin level measured in International Units, and the populations being the age groups (in years) specified below:

```
I :   (1 – 3⁻)      38    5  13  18  54  66  27  73
II :  (3 – 6⁻)      62   30  78  43  45  43  40  64
                    43   32  25  61  41  65  84
III: (6 – 8⁻)       75   74  58  92  38  30  62  62
                    29   82
IV : (8 – 10⁻)      40   82  45  48  59  72  78  99
                    36  100  87  78
```

A preliminary plot of $\bar{X} \pm s$ for each sample, similar to Figure 10.1, revealed no unusual features and no discrepancies among the values of s that could not be attributed to chance. Calculations carried out as in steps 1 to 7 above resulted in Table 10.2.

Table 10.2. Analysis of variance for Example 10.2.

Source of Variation	Sum of Squares	D.F.	Mean Square
Between age groups	5493.61	3	1831.20
Within age groups	18669.37	41	455.35
Total	24162.98	44	

To test the hypothesis of equality of means at, say, the 5% level, we look up $F_{3,41}$ (.05). Since this is not given in the table, we use, as an approximation, $F_{3,40}$ (.05), which is 2.84. Now the ratio $R = MS(between) / MS(within)$ equals 4.02. Since this is larger than 2.84, we reject H_0 at this level.

Note that the null hypothesis would have been accepted at the 1% level, since in that case the significant values of the test statistic are those that are larger than 4.31. The P-value of the statistic is a little over 1%.

10.4. COMPARISONS AMONG MEANS

If the hypothesis of equality of all means is rejected, the next step in the analysis is investigating the reasons for that rejection and deciding which of the k means, if any, are equal. This analysis can also be carried out independently of the outcome of the F ratio test since it studies in more detail the relative values of the population means.

Several different methods have been proposed for such an analysis. We consider here only two: one is a method of comparison by pairs, and the other a method of multiple comparisons.

10.4 a. Comparison by Pairs

Starting with the k sample means, we arrange them by value in ascending order like the following,

$$\overline{X}_{(1)} \leqslant \overline{X}_{(2)} \leqslant \ldots \leqslant \overline{X}_{(k)}$$

where the subscripts refer to the relative values of $\overline{X}$ and are usually different from the original numbering of the populations. Taking the first two, we perform a two-tailed test of the hypothesis that the two population means are equal, using the t-test of Chapter 9 and in particular Formula (9.20) with a modified definition of T_0. If the two means are found significantly different, then $\overline{X}_{(1)}$ must be significantly different from the other larger means as well, and we turn our attention to comparing $\overline{X}_{(2)}$ with those means that are larger than it. If at any stage two means are judged not significantly different, the smaller of the two is compared with all the means appearing to the right of the larger one.

In each of these repetitions of the t-test, the difference between the two sample means is considered significant at level α if it is numerically larger than the quantity

$$D = t(\alpha/2).s\sqrt{\frac{1}{n_1} + \frac{1}{n_2}} \tag{10.1}$$

where t $(\alpha/2)$ is in the right tail of the t distribution with $n-k$ degrees of freedom and exceeded with probability $\alpha/2$, $s^2 = MS(within)$ and is the unbiased estimate of σ^2, n_1 and n_2 are the sizes of the two samples being considered.

If the samples are all of the same size, say n, the critical quantity D defined in (10.1) becomes a common criterion for all pairs and, once calculated, it is used as the same yardstick against which one difference after another is measured. In such cases D is called the *least significant difference* and is given by

$$L.S.D. = t(\alpha/2).s\sqrt{2/n} \ . \tag{10.2}$$

Example 10.3. The means of the four samples in Example 10.2, with the original population numbers as labels, are

I	II	III	IV
36.75	50.40	60.20	68.67

The means are already in ascending order and require no rearrangement. We take α as .05. To calculate D, we need $t_{41}(.025)$. Since our table does not give percentiles for 41 degrees of freedom, we use $t_{40}\,(.025) = 2.021$ as an approximation. This makes

$$D = (43.13)\sqrt{\frac{1}{n_1} + \frac{1}{n_2}} \ .$$

For populations I and II, $n_1 = 8$ and $n_2 = 15$, therefore $D = 18.88$. Since $|\overline{X}_{(1)} - \overline{X}_{(2)}| < 18.88$, the difference is not significant, and we show this by drawing a line below the two means to indicate a connection between them. For populations I and III, $n_1 = 8$ and $n_2 = 10$, therefore $D = 20.46$, and we see that the difference between the sample means is significant. Therefore $\overline{X}_{(1)}$ and $\overline{X}_{(4)}$ are significantly different too. Continuing in the same way, we find:

$\overline{X}_{(2)}$ and $\overline{X}_{(3)}$ are not significantly different,

$\overline{X}_{(2)}$ and $\overline{X}_{(4)}$ are significantly different,

$\overline{X}_{(3)}$ and $\overline{X}_{(4)}$ are not significantly different.

All these relationships are summarized by the lines drawn under the sample means and connecting those with non-significant differences.

As we have seen, this method of comparisons by pairs is easy to apply, whether the sample sizes are equal or not, and the results are easy to interpret. Its weakness lies in the fact that, although P(Error of Type I) for each test is kept no higher than α, the overall probability of rejecting one or another of the series of null hypotheses, while the population means are in fact equal, is a lot larger than α and increases with the number of pairs compared.

10.4 b. Multiple Comparisons

This method is applicable to contrasts among population means. A *contrast* among $\mu_1, \ldots, \mu_k$ is defined as the linear combination

$$L = \sum_{i=1}^{k} c_i \mu_i \qquad \text{where } \sum_{i=1}^{k} c_i = 0;$$

the c_i, some of which are positive and some negative, are chosen in such a way that the joint effect of the combination of means with the positive c_i is balanced against the joint effect of those with the negative c_i, and if the two effects are equal L is zero. For example, if there are five populations of which one is a control and the other 4 are different treatments, a meaningful contrast might compare the control on the one hand with all the treatments put together on the other, and could be written as

$$L = \mu_1 - \frac{1}{4}(\mu_2 + \mu_3 + \mu_4 + \mu_5).$$

The coefficients c_i in this contrast are: $1, -1/4, -1/4, -1/4, -1/4$, which add up to zero as required. In this example, if the treatments are on the average equivalent to the control, then $L = 0$. Notice that the same comparison among the five means can be described equally well by $L = 4\mu_1 - (\mu_2 + \mu_3 + \mu_4 + \mu_5)$ or, for that matter, by any multiple of L.

As another example, we take the difference between μ_1 and μ_5 in the case of the five populations. This difference can be written as

$$L = \mu_1 + 0\mu_2 + 0\mu_3 + 0\mu_4 - \mu_5,$$

so that $c_1 = 1$, $c_5 = -1$ and all the other c_i are zero. It is easy to see that the difference between any two means can be expressed in this way. Therefore the analysis of contrasts includes the analysis of pairs as a special case.

In practice, the choice of contrasts is arbitrary. Some contrasts may be of interest to the investigator from the initial stages of the study, while others may be suggested by the data after the analysis of variance has been carried out. Drori (1976), for example, compared seven dietary treatments in their effect on food intake and fat deposition in male rats. The treatments were as follows:

1— control
2— same as control but with 10 g of NaCl/kg added to food
3— same as control but with 20 g of NaCl/kg added to food
4— same as control but with 30 g of NaCl/kg added to food
5— same as control but with 5 g of NaCl/kg added to drinking water
6— same as control but with 10 g of NaCl/kg added to drinking water
7— same as control but with 15 g of NaCl/kg added to drinking water

If the author had wished to carry out additional analysis by multiple comparisons, it would appear from the plan of the experiment that a contrast such as

$$L_1 = \mu_2 + \mu_3 + \mu_4 - (\mu_5 + \mu_6 + \mu_7),$$

or a contrast such as

$$L_2 = \mu_2 + \mu_3 + \mu_4 + \mu_5 + \mu_6 + \mu_7 - 6\mu_1,$$

or a contrast such as

$$L_3 = 2\mu_4 - (\mu_2 + \mu_3)$$

etc., might be interesting.

If only one or two contrasts among the population means are to be looked into, the analysis is similar to that of comparing pairs of means. In particular, to test the hypothesis that a contrast is zero, H_0: $L = 0$, against a two-sided alternative, one starts out by calculating the estimate of L, which is the corresponding contrast among the sample means, $\Sigma\,c_i\overline{X}_i$. If this estimate is numerically larger than

$$D_L = t\,(\alpha/2).s\sqrt{\Sigma\,c_i^2/n_i},\tag{10.3}$$

H_0 is rejected and L is judged to be different from zero. As before, t has n−k d.f.

Equivalently, one can construct a confidence interval for L, with confidence coefficient 1−α, in the form

$$\Sigma\,c_i\overline{X}_i \pm t\,(\alpha/2).\,s\sqrt{\Sigma\,c_i^2/n_i}\tag{10.4}$$

and reject the null hypothesis at level α if the value of L specified by it, usually zero, is not in the interval.

When several contrasts are tested with the same data, the same problem arises as in the case of comparing pairs, namely that the probability of judging several contrasts different from zero when in fact they are zero is considerable and certainly larger than α. This difficulty is avoided by using a method for multiple comparisons due to Scheffé (1959).

Scheffé's method provides means for constructing a confidence interval for any contrast in such a way that, no matter how many contrasts are estimated, the overall probability that they are simultaneously covered by their respective intervals is a preassigned confidence level, 1−α. In terms of the corresponding two-tailed tests of hypotheses about the contrasts, the method controls the overall probability of erroneously rejecting any of the hypotheses, if the population means are all equal, at a preassigned level α.

To calculate the confidence limits for the contrast $L = \Sigma c_i\mu_i$, we start with its estimate, $\Sigma c_i\overline{X}_i$, and the standard error of the estimate s.$\sqrt{\Sigma c_i^2/n_i}$, where $s^2 = $ MS(within). Let $F_{k-1,n-k}\,(\alpha)$ denote the 100 (1−α) percentile of the F distribution with k−1 and n−k degrees of freedom. Then the confidence limits at level 1−α are

$$\Sigma\,c_i\overline{X}_i \pm \sqrt{(k-1)\,F_{k-1,\,n-k}(\alpha).s.}\sqrt{\Sigma c_i^2/n_i}.\tag{10.5}$$

Note (1).   If all the population means are equal, then all contrasts among those means are zero. This is easy to see for, if the means are all equal to μ, $L = \mu\,\Sigma c_i = 0$. On the other hand, even if several contrasts among the means are zero, the means are not necessarily all equal.

Note (2).   We are usually interested in whether or not a contrast is zero because that expresses a certain balance between two subsets of the populations. However, the testing methods described above are applicable to testing hypotheses about values of contrasts other than zero as well. In general, if the null hypothesis is H_0 : $L = L_0$, the significant values of the estimate of L are those numerically larger than

$$D_L = L_0 + t\,(\alpha/2)\,s\sqrt{\Sigma c_i^2/n_i}.\tag{10.6}$$

which reduces to (10.3) if $L_0 = 0$.

Example 10.4. We return to the results of Example 10.2 (p. 122) and consider the contrasts:

$$L_1 = \mu_2 - \mu_1$$

$$L_2 = 2|\mu_4 - (\mu_1 + \mu_2)$$

$$L_3 = \mu_1 + \mu_3 - \mu_2 - \mu_4.$$

These contrasts were selected purely for illustration and not for any need to investigate them in that problem. For a 95% confidence level, we find $F_{3,41}(.05) = 2.84$. Since $s = 21.34$, all the intervals are of the form: $\Sigma c_i \bar{X}_i \pm 62.29 \sqrt{\Sigma c_i^2 / n_i}$. Substituting the values of n_i and the coefficients c_i in each case, we obtain

$$-13.62 \leqslant L_1 \leqslant 40.92$$
$$5.06 \leqslant L_2 \leqslant 95.32$$
$$-60.65 \leqslant L_3 \leqslant 16.41$$

Of the three contrasts considered, only the second appears to be significantly different from zero. Other contrasts among the four means could have been considered as well, and our confidence in the entire set of such conslusions is 95%.

10.5. TRANSFORMATIONS

Although the basic model for the analysis of variance requires that the observations come from normal populations with equal variances, these requirements are rarely met in practice, and the extent to which they are violated affects the validity of the subsequent inference. It is therefore important for the investigator to be able to decide whether the assumptions are at least approximately satisfied in his problem and, if they are not, to know what can be done to remedy the situation. Hence, before carrying out any calculations, he must (a) examine the data for marked departures from the model and, if necessary, (b) apply an appropriate transformation to the data to bring it more in line with the basic assumptions.

(a). The two assumptions, that of normality and that of equal variances, need not be checked separately, as it usually turns out that when one of these assumptions is violated so is the other. The reason is that, while the variance of a normal population is in no way related to the mean, in many non-normal populations the variance is a well-defined function of the mean. For example, in the binomial population, the mean is np and the variance is $np(1-p)$; in a Poisson population, the mean and variance are equal; and in a Chi-square population the variance is twice the mean. Therefore, if our populations are not normal a lack of equality among the population means very likely carries with it a lack of equality among the population variances. For normal populations, it is quite possible for the variances to be equal and for the means to be very different from each other.

A simple way to check on the equality of the population variances is to calculate the sample variances (or standard deviations) and display their values graphically with the values of the sample means, as was done in Figure 10.1, or in a simple plot of variance against mean as in Figure 10.3. If the graph suggests a functional relation between sample mean and variance, then this relation very likely exists between population mean and variance, and thus the populations from which the samples were taken may very well be non-normal.

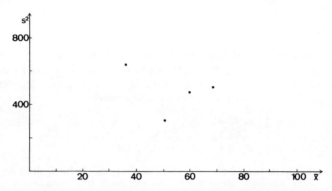

FIG. 10.3.   Sample means and variances from data in Example 10.2

(b). When a study of sample means and variances reveals a marked departure from the model, the observations may be transformed into a new set to which the methods of the previous sections of this chapter are better suited. Three commonly used transformations are the following:

(i) *The Logarithmic Transformation.* If the graph of sample variances against sample means suggests a relation of the form

$$s^2 = (a\ constant).(\overline{X^2}),$$

replace each observation X by its logarithm to the base 10,

$$Y = \log_{10}X; \tag{10.7}$$

or, if some X values are zero, by $Y = \log_{10}(X + 1)$.

(ii) *The Square Root Transformation.* If the relation is of the form

$$s^2 = (a\ constant).(\overline{X}),$$

replace each X by its square root,

$$Y = \sqrt{X} \tag{10.8}$$

or, if the X's are very close to zero, by the square root of $(X + 1/2)$. This relation is found in data from Poisson populations, where the variance is equal to the mean.

(iii) *The Angular Transformation.* If the observations are counts of a binomial nature, and $\hat{p}$ is the observed proportion, replace $\hat{p}$ by

$$\theta = \arcsin \sqrt{\hat{p}}, \tag{10.9}$$

which is the principal angle (in degrees or radians) whose sine is the square root of $\hat{p}$. This transformation needs either a combination of square root and arcsin tables or function keys on the calculator, or a special table giving the transformed value directly, such as Table X of Fisher and Yates (1974).

Note (1). All calculations in the analysis of variance and in constructing confidence intervals and testing hypotheses are done with the transformed variables. However, one may wish at the conclusion of the analysis to quote some results in the original scale, such as the estimates of the means and the confidence limits. Each of these quantities is obtained by applying the inverse transformation to the calculated statistic. This is illustrated in Example 10.7.

Note (2). Each of the three given transformations, (10.7), (10.8) and (10.9), has the effect of removing a dependence between the population mean and variance that existed in the untransformed data, and was derived from a knowledge of that relationship. It is therefore reasonable to expect that other types of dependence would call for other transformations. This is indeed the case, and the appropriate transformation can usually be derived mathematically. A number of useful transformations, which include the ones mentioned above, were given by Bartlett (1947) and are reproduced in several statistics books dealing with the design and analysis of experiments (see, for instance, Kempthorne (1952, p. 156)).

The following examples, in each of which the data was extracted from a larger set of observations, will serve to illustrate the use of transformations in one-way analysis of variance problems. Each of these sets of data appears in the cited publication in connection with problems other than the equality of population means and, we presume, were not collected for this type of analysis. However, since other experiments along similar lines may be planned for the purpose of comparing means, we consider these data sets suitable as illustrations for the methods of this section.

Example 10.5. Using data from the Regional Poisoning Treatment Center of the Royal Infirmary at Edinburgh, Duffy (1977) studied the frequency distribution of parasuicides per year in four different groups of persons: A – men, without previous episodes, B – women, without previous episodes, C – men, repeaters, and D – women, repeaters. We let these groups define four populations, and we take as our variable the total number of parasuicides in a population per year. From the five-year record for each group, we took a sample of 3 observations on this variable. These observations, together with the calculated $\overline{X}$ and s^2 from each sample, are shown in Table 10.3(a). Figure 10.4(a) shows a plot of the four pairs $(\overline{X}, s^2)$ which suggests that the relation between the variance and the mean can be well described by the line $s^2 = $ (a constant).$(\overline{X})$, and therefore the square root transformation is indicated. The transformed data is shown in Table 10.3(b), and Figure 10.4(b) shows a plot of the sample variance against sample mean in the transformed scale.

Table 10.3. Original and transformed data from Example 10.5.

(a)

	A	B	C	D
	163	344	134	194
	200	399	151	236
	181	386	166	242
$\overline{X}$:	181.3	376.3	150.3	224.0
s^2 :	342.2	826.3	256.3	684.0

(b)

	A	B	C	D
	12.77	18.55	11.58	13.93
	14.14	19.97	12.29	15.36
	13.45	19.65	12.88	15.56
$\overline{X}$:	13.45	19.39	12.25	14.95
s^2 :	.47	.55	.42	.79

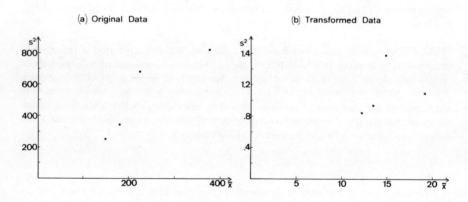

FIG. 10.4. Sample means and variances from Example 10.5 ·

Example 10.6. In this example, we use observations taken by Sweatman and Koussa (1968) on the metabolic rate (in $\mu l\ O_2/mg/hr$) of female ticks under different temperature conditions. Taking four different temperature groups as four populations, we calculated $\overline{X}$ and s^2 from each sample, and plotted the 4 points as in Figure 10.5(a). Since the graph suggested a quadratic relation between the mean and variance $(s^2 = (\text{constant})\ (\overline{X}^2)\ )$ the logarithmic transformation was applied to the data. A plot of the 4 points, each representing the mean and variance of a transformed sample, is shown in Figure 10.5(b) and demonstrates a considerable stabilization in the variances as a result of the transformation.

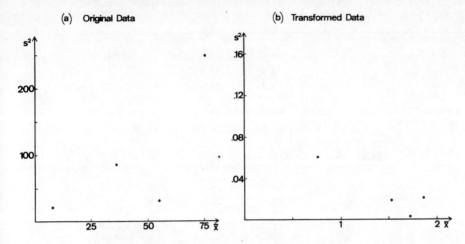

FIG. 10.5. Sample means and variances from Example 10.6

Example 10.7. Mertz and Davies (1968) report the result of an investigation of cannibalism in flour beetles under different predator-to-prey densities. Their data appear as counts of surviving prey in each of five blocks, with the initial numbers of predators and prey also given. For our illustration, we use some of the counts corresponding to 96 predators per block and take the variable as the percentage surviving at the termination of the observation period. The 3 different populations are distinguished by different predator-to-prey ratio. This data is clearly of the binomial type, and the arcsin transformation seems appropriate. In Table 10.4, we give the original and transformed data (where the transformation was done with the aid of Table X of Fisher and Yates (1974)), and then use the latter for the usual analysis of variance calculations. The analysis of variance table appears at the bottom of Table 10.4, and is followed by the calculation of a confidence interval.

We now construct a confidence interval for the difference between the mean survival percentages corresponding to populations II and III, so that in terms of Formula (10.4) $c_1 = 0$, $c_3 = 1$ and $c_2 = -1$. Let $\alpha = .10$, then $t_{12}(.05) = 1.782$. We have $n_2 = n_3 = 5$ and, from the MS(within), $s = 4.10$. This yields the interval 5.20 ± 4.62 or $(.58, 9.82)$ in the transformed scale. Using the angular transformation table in the opposite direction, we find that when $\arcsin \sqrt{\hat{p}} = .58$, $\hat{p} = .0001$, and when $\arcsin \sqrt{\hat{p}} = 9.82$, $\hat{p} = .0291$. Therefore the 90% confidence interval for the difference between the two percentages is

$$0.01 \leqslant 100\, p_1 - 100\, p_2 \leqslant 2.91.$$

Table 10.4. Data from Example 10.7
(a) Original and (b) transformed (to nearest integer)

(a)

	I	II	III
	9.4	18.8	27.8
	18.8	14.1	21.9
	7.3	12.0	22.2
	8.3	24.5	20.8
	9.4	21.4	35.4
$\bar{X}$:	10.64	18.16	25.62
s^2 :	21.57	26.38	37.29

(b)

	I	II	III
	18	26	32
	26	22	28
	16	20	28
	17	30	27
	18	28	37
$\bar{X}$:	19	25.2	30.4
s^2 :	16	17.2	17.3

Analysis of Variance (transformed data)

Source	Sum of Squares	d.f.	Mean Square
Between ratios	325.73	2	162.87
Within ratios	202.00	12	16.83
Total	527.73	14	

REFERENCES

Bartlett, M.S. (1947). The use of transformations. Biometrics, journal of The Biometric Society, *3*, 39-52.

Drori, D. (1976). The effect of sodium chloride ingestion on food intake and on fat deposition in male rats. Br. J. Nutr. *35*, 195-199. Cambridge University Press, Cambridge, England.

Duffy, J.C. (1977). Frequency distribution of hospital-referred parasuicidal episodes in Edinburgh. Br. J. prev. soc. Med. *31*, 109-115.

Feisal, K.A., Eckstein, J.W., Horsley, A.W., and Keasling, H.H. (1961). Effects of chlorothiazide on forearm vascular responses to norepinephrine. J. appl. Physiol. *16*, 549-552.

Fisher, R.A. and Yates, F. (1974). *Statistical Tables for Biological, Agricultural and Medical Research,* 6th ed., Longman Group Ltd., London.

Kemphtorne, O. (1952). *The Design and Analysis of Experiments.* Wiley, New York.

Mertz, D.B. and Davies, R.B. (1968). Cannibalism of the pupal stage by adult flour beetles: an experiment and a stochastic model. Biometrics, journal of The Biometric Society, *24*, 247-275.

Scheffé , H. (1959). *The Analysis of Vairance.* Wiley, New York.

Sweatman, G.K. and Koussa, M.G. (1968). Comparative changes in external respiration rates of engorged *Rhipicephalus sanguineus* female ticks with age and oviposition in different physical environments. J. Parasit. *54*, 641-656.

CHAPTER 11

Comparing Standard Deviations

11.1. INTRODUCTION

In comparing two or more means from independent samples, the usual assumption is that the standard deviations (or variances) of the populations compared are equal. A graphical method for checking on such an assumption in several independent samples was given in Section 10.5 in connection with the analysis of variance technique. This chapter contains two tests of the hypothesis that the population variances are equal, an exact test for the case of two populations, and an approximate test for more than two. Both tests are based on the assumption that the observations come from normal populations. Needless to say, testing the equality of variances may itself be the main object of the investigation and is not necessarily restricted to being a side issue in the comparison of means.

The variability in different populations can also be compared by means of a simple descriptive statistic, called the sample *coefficient of variation,* and defined as the ratio of sample standard deviation to sample mean, or

$$V = s/\overline{X} \quad . \tag{11.1}$$

The coefficient of variation is independent of the units in which the observations are made, and is thus useful when comparing different characteristics in the same group or the same characteristic in disparate groups. As an example of the former, consider a group of adults with varying heights, weights and blood pressures; the variability of each of these characteristics can best be compared with those of the others through a comparison of the coefficients of variation. As an example of the other use, take the comparison of the variability of weight gains of guinea pigs on a high protein diet and weight gains of humans on a high protein diet; the observations on the two groups are so different that a comparison of the standard deviations would be meaningless.

The coefficient of variation is usually stated as a percentage.

11.2. COMPARING TWO STANDARD DEVIATIONS. The F Test

Let σ_1 and σ_2 be the standard deviations of two normal populations and suppose that the problem is to test their equality or, more generally, to find out to what extent, if any, they differ in magnitude. This problem can be more conveniently expressed in terms of a single parameter, σ_1^2 / σ_2^2, which is the ratio of the two population variances. It is easy to see that this parameter is equal to 1 when the two standard deviations are equal and, whether or not they are equal, it can serve as a measure of their relative sizes.

Let a sample of size n_1 be taken from the first population and a sample of size n_2 from the second, and let s_1^2 and s_2^2, respectively, be the sample variances, each calculated in the usual way by Formula (7.1). Then the ratio of the population variances can be estimated by the corresponding ratio

$$R = s_1^2 / s_2^2. \tag{11.2}$$

This statistic, which may be calculated by means of Program DEVS1 of Chapter 18, will be used to construct confidence intervals and tests of hypotheses concerning the parameter σ_1^2 / σ_2^2. As the reader can verify, these methods are all based on the fact that

(a) in each sample, the quantity $(n-1)s^2/\sigma^2$ has a χ^2_{n-1} distribution, and

(b) the ratio of the two independent variables,

$$\frac{s_1^2}{\sigma_1^2} \Big/ \frac{s_2^2}{\sigma_2^2} \, ,$$

has an $F_{n_1-1, \, n_2-1}$ distribution (see Section 4.4).

To apply each of the following methods, one needs to consult Table V in the Appendix or a similar table of the F-distribution for the required percentiles. We recall that Table V gives only two percentiles in the right tail for each (n_1-1, n_2-1) combination, in particular the percentile $F_{n_1-1, \, n_2-1}(\alpha)$, which is exceeded with probability α, for $\alpha = .01$ and $.05$. We also recall that the corresponding percentile in the left tail, namely $F_{n_1-1, \, n_2-1}(1-\alpha)$, can be obtained by reversing the order of the degrees of freedom, looking up the percentile for that reversed order, and then taking the reciprocal. In other words,

$$F_{n_1-1, \, n_2-1}(1-\alpha) = \frac{1}{F_{n_2-1, \, n_1-1}(\alpha)} \, .$$

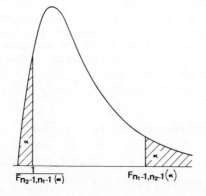

FIG. 11.1. Two percentiles of the F-distribution with (n_1-1, n_2-1) d.f.

(i) *A confidence interval* for σ_1^2/σ_2^2 at level $1-\alpha$. This is given by

$$\frac{R}{F_{n_1-1,\,n_2-1}(\alpha/2)} \leqslant \frac{\sigma_1^2}{\sigma_2^2} \leqslant R.\,F_{n_2-1,\,n_1-1}\,(\alpha/2). \tag{11.3}$$

The percentiles in Table V correspond to $\alpha/2 = .01$ or $.05$, and therefore only confidence levels of 98% or 90% are possible to obtain from this table. More extensive tables are needed for other confidence levels.

(ii) *A two-tailed test of the hypothesis* $H_0 : \sigma_1^2 / \sigma_2^2 = k$ at significance level α. For $k = 1$, this is a test of-equality of the two variances. The test statistic is R and its significant values, at level α, are

$$R > k\,F_{n_1-1,\,n_2-1}\,(\alpha/2)$$

$$\tag{11.4}$$

$$\text{or} \quad R < \frac{k}{F_{n_2-1,\,n_1-1}\,(\alpha/2)}$$

An equivalent test is to construct a confidence interval at confidence level $1-\alpha$ and reject the null hypothesis H_0 if the number k is not in the interval.

For this test, Table V can be used if α is taken as $.02$ or $.10$.

(iii) *A one-tailed test* of the hypothesis $H_0 : \sigma_1^2/\sigma_2^2 = k$ against $H_R : \sigma_1^2/\sigma_2^2 > k$ at significance level α. In this case, the significant values of the test statistic are

$$R > k.\,F_{n_1-1,\,n_2-1}\,(\alpha),$$

$$\tag{11.5}$$

and Table V can be used if α is taken as $.01$ or $.05$.

This test is appropriate when $\cdot\sigma_1^2$ is suspected of being larger than σ_2^2 so $H_0 : \sigma_1^2/\sigma_2^2 = 1$ is tested against $H_R : \sigma_1^2/\sigma_2^2 > 1$. If the situation is such that σ_1^2 is suspected of being *smaller* than σ_2^2, one simply relabels the populations to make the potentially larger variance that of the first population.

Example 11.1. A sample of 7 systolic blood pressure readings for individuals in one age group had a standard deviation of 10.41, and a sample of 14 readings from another age group had a standard deviation of 13.75 (Abou-Daoud, 1978). Is systolic blood pressure significantly more variable in the second group than in the first, or could this discrepancy between the two sample standard deviations have arisen by chance in two samples having the same population standard deviation?

We first test the hypothesis $H_0 : \sigma_1^2/\sigma_2^2 = 1$ against $H_R : \sigma_1^2/\sigma_2^2 > 1$ at the 5% level, after labelling the populations so that the population suspected of being more variable is population No. 1. Then, $n_1 = 14$ and $n_2 = 7$, and we look up $F_{13,6}(.05)$ in Table V. Interpolating between 12 and 15 for the degrees of freedom in the sum of the squares of the numerator, we get $F_{13,6}(.05) = 3.98$. Therefore the significant values of $R = s_1^2/s_2^2$ are, by (11.5), those larger than 3.98. But $R = (13.75)^2/(10.41)^2 = 1.745$, which is smaller than 3.98. Therefore we accept the hypothesis tested, at the 5% level.

To construct a 90% confidence interval for the ratio σ_1^2/σ_2^2, we find $F_{6,13}(.05) = 2.92$. This is substituted in (11.3), together with the value of $F_{13,6}(.05)$ already obtained and the observed value of R, resulting in the interval

$$\frac{1.745}{3.98} \leqslant \frac{\sigma_1^2}{\sigma_1^2} \leqslant (1.745)(2.92)$$

or $0.44 \leqslant \dfrac{\sigma_1^2}{\sigma_2^2} \leqslant 5.09.$

11.3. SEVERAL STANDARD DEVIATIONS .   Bartlett's Test

For testing the hypothesis that the standard deviations of k normal populations (k > 2) are equal, we can use the following approximate test due to Bartlett (1937):

1) For each sample of size n_i , calculate the sample variance s_i^2.

2) Combine the sample variances as in the pooled estimate of a common variance,

$$\overline{s}^2 = \frac{\sum\limits_{i=1}^{k} (n_i-1)\, s_i^2}{\sum\limits_{i=1}^{k} (n_i-1)} \, .$$

3) Calculate $M = 2.303\ (\log \overline{s}^2\ \Sigma\ (n_i-1) - \Sigma\ (n_i-1) \log s_i^2)$, (logarithm to base 10).

4) Calculate a scaling constant

$$C = 1 + \frac{1}{3(k-1)}\ [\ \Sigma \frac{1}{n_i-1} - \frac{1}{\Sigma(n_i-1)}\ ]$$

which is usually close to 1.

5) Calculate the test statistic M/C. This has approximately a Chi-Square distribution with k−1 degrees of freedom.

6) The significant values of M/C are given by

$$M/C\ >\ \chi^2{}_{k-1}(\alpha)\ ,   \tag{11.6}$$

where $\chi^2{}_{k-1}(\alpha)$ is the 100 $(1-\alpha)$ percentile of the Chi-square distribution with k−1 degrees of freedom, as shown in Figure 11.2. This test statistic may also be calculated by means of Program DEVS2 of Chapter 18.

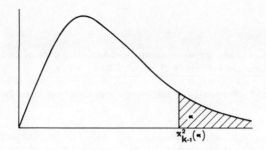

FIG. 11.2. Upper tail percentile of the Chi-square distribution
with $k-1$ d.f.

This test is suitable for fairly large samples, but 5 or more observations per sample have been found adequate. For smaller samples, a more accurate test is provided in a special table of significant values of the statistic M which can be found in the first volume of the Biometrika Tables (Pearson and Hartley, 1966).

Example 11.2. Irving *et al* (1974) counted limb motor neurones in the right and left sides of segments of the lumbosacral cord and commented on the higher variability in some of the segments. We use their 11 counts for each of eight segments to test the hypothesis that the variations in the number of neurones are the same in all 8 sections. Here, $k = 8$ and $n_i - 1 = 10$ for all i. We have calculated the sample variances and their logarithms as follows:—

s^2 : 80124   787882   534183   458031   348772   397184   502239   490176

$\log s^2$:   4.90   5.90   5.73   5.66   5.54   5.60   5.70   5.69

This gives us $\bar{s}^{-2} = 449824$ and $\log \bar{s}^{-2} = 5.65$.

Therefore $M = (2.303) ((5.65) (80) - (10) (44.72))$

            $= 11.05$

and $C = 1.0375$, so that $M/C = 10.65$.

Let $\alpha = .05$, then the significant values of the test statistic are those that exceed $\chi^2_7(.05) = 14.07$. We therefore accept the hypothesis.

Note: As mentioned earlier, both the F test and Bartlett's test assume a normal distribution for the variable. If the distribution is very far from normal, the tests may have a larger or a smaller probability of rejecting a true hypothesis than the preassigned level α, depending on the actual distribution in the population. It is therefore advisable, whenever possible, to inquire into the normality of the parent population before applying these tests. Some methods for testing normality will be given in Chapter 15.

REFERENCES

Abou-Daoud, K.T. (1978). *personal communication.* Department of Epidemiology and Biostatistics, American University of Beirut, Beirut, Lebanon.

Bartlett, M.S. (1937). Properties of sufficiency and statistical tests. Proc. R. Soc. A *160*, 268-282.

Irving, D., Rebeiz, J.J., and Tomlinson, B.E. (1974). The numbers of limb motor neurones in the individual segments of the human lumbosacral spinal cord. J. Neurol. Sci. *21*, 203-212.

Pearson, E.S. and Hartley, H.O. (editors) (1966). *Biometrika Tables for Statisticans*, vol. I, 3rd ed., Cambridge University Press, Cambridge, England.

CHAPTER 12
Comparing Proportions

12.1. PROPORTIONS IN TWO INDEPENDENT SAMPLES

Experiments designed for comparing proportions in two independent samples are very common. There are comparisons of cancer incidence in smokers and non-smokers, comparisons of survival rates following two different treatments, comparisons of fractions responding favourably to treatment among men and women, etc. In each case, n_1 observations on a dichotomous variable are taken from one population, and the number observed to belong to the category of interest (call it category S) is denoted by X_1; quite independently, n_2 observations are taken on the same variable from the other population, and the number belonging to S among them is denoted by X_2. Then the outcome of the experiment is summarized as in the following table:

	Sample I	Sample II
Number in S	X_1	X_2
Number not in S	$n_1 - X_1$	$n_2 - X_2$
Total number	n_1	n_2

The problem is whether the proportion of observations belonging to the special category S is the same in the two populations and, if it is not, about how different are the two proportions?

The essential components of the above table are the four counts $X_1, X_2, n_1 - X_1$ and $n_2 - X_2$ appearing in two rows and two columns. Such an arrangement is called a *two by two table*, and written briefly as 2 x 2.

Let the population proportions be denoted, respectively, by p_1 and p_2. As we have seen in the case of one dichotomous population (Chapter 6), these unknown proportions can be estimated by the corresponding sample proportions,

$$\hat{p}_1 = \frac{X_1}{n_1} \quad \text{and} \quad \hat{p}_2 = \frac{X_2}{n_2},$$

each of which is approximately normally distributed — unless it is calculated from a very small sample.

12.1 a. Confidence intervals for the difference $p_1 - p_2$

For a confidence interval at level $1-\alpha$, we calculate the estimate $\hat{p}_1 - \hat{p}_2$ and its standard error,

$$\text{estimated S.E. } (\hat{p}_1 - \hat{p}_2) = \sqrt{\frac{X_1(n_1 - X_1)}{n_1^3} + \frac{X_2(n_2 - X_2)}{n_2^3}}$$

and, for a total area of α in the two tails, we look up $z(\alpha/2)$ in the table of the normal distribution. By analogy with Formula (6.3), the confidence interval has the limits

$$(\hat{p}_1 - \hat{p}_2) \pm z(\alpha/2) \sqrt{\frac{X_1(n_1 - X_1)}{n_1^3} + \frac{X_2(n_2 - X_2)}{n_2^3}}. \qquad (12.1)$$

The corresponding program in Chapter 18 is Program PROP3.

Unlike the interval in Formula (6.3), this interval does not contain a correction for continuity. Some authors recommend that X_1 and X_2 be corrected by half a unit each before calculating $\hat{p}_1$ and $\hat{p}_2$, but the correction is likely to be negligible after the subtraction and would complicate the formula.

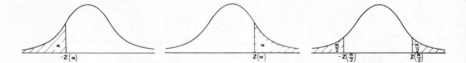

FIG. 12.1.   Percentiles of the standard normal distribution

12.1 b. Testing the hypothesis $H_0 : p_1 = p_2$

This hypothesis can be expressed as $H_0 : p_1 - p_2 = 0$. Again, the tests are based on the statistic $\hat{p}_1 - \hat{p}_2$. Under H_0, this statistic has zero mean and standard error equal to $[p(1-p)/n_1 + p(1-p)/n_2]^{1/2}$, where p is the *common* value of p_1 and p_2. To estimate this common p, we use the pooled estimate,

$$\hat{p} = \frac{X_1 + X_2}{n_1 + n_2}.$$

In this notation, the test statistic, standardized when $p_1 = p_2$, is

$$Z_0 = \frac{\dfrac{X_1}{n_1} - \dfrac{X_2}{n_2} - 0}{[\hat{p}(1-\hat{p}) \, (\dfrac{1}{n_1} + \dfrac{1}{n_2})]^{1/2}} \qquad (12.2)$$

By analogy with the one-sample case, if the significance level is α, the significant values of Z_0 in the three different testing situations are as follows:

(i) For testing $H_0 : p_1 - p_2 \leqslant 0$ against $H_R : p_1 - p_2 > 0$,
$$Z_0 > z\,(\alpha). \qquad (12.3)$$
(ii) For testing $H_0 : p_1 - p_2 \geqslant 0$ against $H_L : p_1 - p_2 < 0$,
$$Z_0 < -z\,(\alpha). \qquad (12.4)$$
(iii) For testing $H_0 : p_1 - p_2 = 0$ against $H_T : p_1 - p_2 \neq 0$.
$$|Z_0| > z\,(\alpha/2). \qquad (12.5)$$

12.1 c. The Chi-square test

The two-tailed test in (iii) above has an alternative method of calculation which does not call for a prior estimation of the common p. The test statistic can be evaluated directly from the entries in the 2 x 2 table. Denote the four frequencies in the table by a, b, c, and d, and calculate the row and column totals as in the following array:

a	b	a + b
c	d	c + d
a + c	b + d	N

With this notation, calculate the statistic

$$Y = \frac{(\,|ad - bc| - N/2)^2 \; N}{(a + b)(c + d)(a + c)(b + d)} , \qquad (12.6)$$

which can also be obtained by means of Program CHIS2 (Chapter 18).

If H_0 is true, this statistic has approximately a Chi-square distribution with 1 degree of freedom. If $p_1 \neq p_2$, Y tends to be larger. Therefore, at significance level α, its significant values are

$$Y > \chi_1^2\,(\alpha). \qquad (12.7)$$

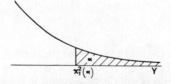

FIG. 12.2. Upper percentile of the Chi-square distribution with 1 d.f.

Note (1). All of the methods given above are based on the normal approximation to the binomial distribution and are therefore *large sample methods*, which are not very reliable when the sample sizes are small. If n_1 and n_2 are small ($\leqslant 15$), *exact* one-tailed and two-tailed tests of H_0 can be carried out with the aid of a special table (see Pearson and Hartley, 1966, Table 38).

Note (2). Formula (12.6) is sometimes given without the subtraction of the term $N/2$ in the numerator. This term, known as *Yates' correction for continuity,* has been found to improve the performance of this approximate test, particularly when the sample sizes are not very large. When this term is dropped from the formula, the corresponding program in Chapter 18 is Program CHIS1.

If the correction for continuity is ignored, the rules given by (12.7) and (12.5) become identical, for it can be shown that the "uncorrected" statistic Y is the square of Z_0 as defined in (12.2), and therefore (12.7) can be written as $Z_0^2 > \chi_1^2 (\alpha)$ or, equivalently, as $|Z_0| > \sqrt{\chi_1^2(\alpha)}$. In (12.5), the rule is expressed in terms of the percentile $z(\alpha/2)$, but $[z(\alpha/2)]^2 = \chi_1^2(\alpha)$ because, if the probability is $\alpha/2$ that a standard normal variable is larger than a certain positive number, the probability is twice $\alpha/2$ (or α) that its square is larger than the square of that number. This fact is demonstrated in Figure 12.3.

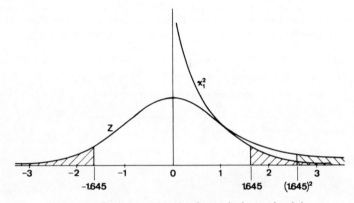

FIG. 12.3. Equivalent tests using the standard normal and the Chi-square distribution with 1 d.f.

Note (3). 2 x 2 tables may result from a different type of experiment than the one considered in this section, yet the mechanics of carrying out the test of the appropriate null hypothesis are precisely the same in both cases. In Chapter 13 we consider such tables as well as ones with several rows and columns, of which the 2 x 2 table is a special case.

Example 12.1. Lamoureux *et al* (1976) studied the immunological systems of 23 multiple sclerosis (MS) patients and 23 controls, and compared the occurrence of certain infections in the medical histories of the two groups. In the case of tonsillectomy, their findings were

	MS patients	Controls	Both
Tonsillectomy	16	9	25
No Tonsillectomy	7	14	21
Total	23	23	46

(i) A 90% confidence interval for the difference between the proportions of tonsillectomy in the history of the two populations is, by (12.1),

$$\frac{16}{23} - \frac{9}{23} \pm z(.05) \sqrt{\frac{(16)(7)}{23^3} + \frac{(9)(14)}{23^3}}$$

or $.30 \pm .23$,   that is $.07 \leqslant p_1 - p_2 \leqslant .53$.

(ii) To test $H_0 : p_1 = p_2$ against $H_R : p_1 > p_2$, at the 5% level, we calculate the common estimate $\hat{p} = 25/46 = .54$ and apply the rule in (12.3). Here $Z_0 = .304/.147 = 2.07$. Since $z(.05) = 1.645$, we reject H_0 at this level.

(iii) To test $H_0 : p_1 = p_2$ against $H_T : p_1 \neq p_2$ at the 10% level, we use Formula (12.6) and calculate $Y = 3.15$. Corresponding to $\alpha = .10$, we find $\chi_1^2(.10) = 2.71$. Since $3.15 > 2.71$, we reject H_0 at this level. We observe, in connection with Note (2), that $(1.645)^2 = 2.71$.

12.2. PROPORTIONS IN TWO MATCHED SAMPLES

Two samples are matched (or paired) when every observation in the first sample is related to a single observation in the second. The two observations may, for example, be taken under the same conditions in two different groups or on the same subject under two different treatments. The purpose of pairing is to minimize the effect of factors other than those that distinguish the two populations.

Paired samples with numerical observations were discussed in Chapter 9. The difference here is that the observed variable is of the dichotomous type, so that every pair of observations consists of two statements, the first asserting whether or not the special category has been observed in the first sample, and the second making a similar assertion about the second sample. Denoting the occurrence of the special category by S and its nonoccurrence by F, we see that every pair of observations must be one of the four types:

   (S,S), (S,F), (F,S), or (F,F).

For example, suppose that we are interested in the smoking habits of the two parents of teenagers who are themselves smokers, and that we wish to compare the proportion of heavy smokers among the fathers with the proportion of heavy smokers among the mothers. The observations on each teenager in the sample would be an ordered pair of statements, the first concerning the father and the second concerning the mother, and each being denoted by S if that parent was a heavy smoker and by F if the parent was not a heavy smoker.

Let the sample consist of n pairs, and consider the problem of testing the hypothesis

$$H_0 : p_1 = p_2$$

against a one-sided or a two-sided alternative on the basis of these observations. As before, p_1 and p_2 are the proportions of the special category in the two populations.

It should be clear that, of the four types of pairs in the set of observations, the ones in which the two observations are identical (namely the pairs of type (S,S) and (F,F)) provide no information on any differences that may exist between the two proportions. Therefore the test statistic will be based on pairs of the types (S,F) or (F,S) only. Let the sample contain r_1 of the former and r_2 of the latter type. Then, if H_0 is true, we would expect r_1 and r_2 to be equal; if $p_1 > p_2$, we would expect r_1 to be larger than r_2, and if $p_1 < p_2$ we would expect it to be smaller. Since the decision is based on the *relative* values of r_1 and r_2, we consider $r_1 + r_2$ fixed and take one of them, say r_1, as the test statistic. Since this statistic is a count of pairs of type (S,F) out of a fixed number $r_1 + r_2$ of pairs, it is a binomial variable with parameters $(r_1 + r_2, \pi)$, where π is the proportion of (S,F) pairs among all possible pairs of the two types. Since $\pi = .5$ if H_0 is true and $> .5$ or $< .5$ if the type (S,F) is more likely or less likely, respectively, than the other type, the problem   reduces to the testing problem of Section 6.5, with r_1 replacing X, $r_1 + r_2$ replacing n, and .5 replacing p_0 of that section.

When $r_1 + r_2 \geqslant 10$, the normal approximation to the binomial distribution is adequate, and the formulas of Section 6.5 simplify to the following rules:

1) Calculate the standardized statistic r_1 under H_0. This is

$$Z_0 = \frac{r_1 - r_2 - 1}{\sqrt{r_1 + r_2}} , \qquad (12.8)$$

where the term -1 represents correction for continuity;

2)   (i) For testing $H_0 : p_1 = p_2$ against $H_R : p_1 > p_2$ at significance level α, the significant values of Z_0 are

$$Z_0 > z(\alpha) ;$$

(ii) For testing H_0 against $H_L : p_1 < p_2$, the significant values are

$$Z_0 < -z(\alpha);$$

(iii) For testing H_0 against $H_T : p_1 \neq p_2$, the signifcant values are

$$|Z_0| > z (\alpha/2).$$

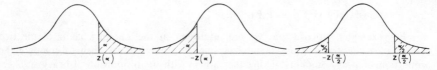

FIG. 12.4. Percentiles of the standard normal distribution

Example 12.2. As an illustration for a linear structural relationships model for quantitative variables, Barnett (1969) used readings of vital capacity for 72 patients on four combinations of instruments and operatives. The first set of readings, y_0 , was taken by a skilled operative on a standard instrument, and two other readings, y_2 and y_3, were taken by skilled and unskilled operatives on an experimental instrument. We consider the skilled and unskilled readings on the experimental instrument as the two groups of interest, and apply the methods of this section to Barnett's data in terms of a dichotomous variable. This variable we define in such a way that it occurs whenever a reading is larger than that obtained by a skilled operative on the standard instrument. Thus each of the 144 original readings of y_2 and y_3 is replaced by S if it exceeds y_0 and by F if it does not.

To test the hypothesis that the proportion of higher readings is the same in both groups, against the two-sided alternative, at the 5% significance level, we obtain from the data the following counts:

number of pairs of type (S,S) = 19
number of pairs of type (S,F) = 9
number of pairs of type (F,S) = 5
number of pairs of type (F,F) = 38.

Thus $r_1 = 9$, $r_2 = 5$, and $z_0 = (9\text{-}5\text{-}1)/\sqrt{14} = .80$. Since $z(.025) = 1.96$, and $|z_0| < 1.96$, we accept the null hypothesis that the two proportions are equal at this level. In fact, by calculating the P-value of Z_0 (which is the probability of observing .80 or a more extreme value of Z_0 when H_0 is true) we find it to be .4238, which implies that such an outcome is quite likely under the null hypothesis.
We observe that this test accomplishes only what it sets out to accomplish with this data, namely a comparison between the proportions of high readings in the two groups. It does not compare the readings on the experimental instrument with y_0 readings in general, and neither does it test the accuracy of the readings on the experimental instrument.

12.3. SEVERAL PROPORTIONS

We now consider independent samples taken from k dichotomous populations $(k > 2)$ for the purpose of testing the equality of all k population proportions. This problem is an extension of the one discussed in Section 12.1, and the calculations required in its analysis are fairly simple. An extension of the equality of proportions problem in matched samples, which is more complicated, will not be considered in this book. An elementary account of a test for such a hypothesis, due to Cochran (1950), can be found in Sokal and Rohlf (1969), where the k proportions are referred to as "corelated".

Consider a dichotomous variable, denoting its occurrence in the special category by S and its absence by F, and let p_i be the proportion of elements of type S in the ith population $(i = 1, \ldots, k)$. Let k samples of sizes $n_1, \ldots, n_k$, respectively, be taken from the k populations, each independently of the others, and let X_i be the number of observations of type S in the ith sample, $i = 1, \ldots, k$. Then the set of observations can be summarized in a 2 x k table like the following, in which row totals and column totals are also indicated, with ΣX_i denoted by X and Σn_i by n.

Sample	1	2	...	k	All
Number of S observations	X_1	X_2	...	X_k	X
Number of F observations	$n_1 - X_1$	$n_2 - X_2$	...	$n_k - X_k$	$n - X$
Total	n_1	n_2	...	n_k	n

We use these observations in testing the hypothesis

$$H_0 : p_1 = p_2 = \ldots = p_k$$

against the very general alternative that they are not all equal. To carry out the test, we first figure out what frequencies of S and F would be expected in each sample if H_0 were true, and then we compare those expected frequencies with the observed frequencies that appear in the 2 x k table. If the discrepancy between expected and observed frequencies is mild enough to be attributed to chance fluctuations in samples from identical populations, we accept H_0; if the discrepancy is too large, we reject it. A measure of this discrepancy, which is our test statistic, will be defined below in terms of the expected and observed frequencies:

1) For any cell in the table, denote the observed frequency by the letter O. We can calculate the corresponding expected frequency, E, by the formula

$$E = (\text{row total}) (\text{column total})/n, \tag{12.9}$$

where the row and column are the ones in which that particular cell appears. For example, corresponding to an observed frequency $O = X_2$, the expected frequency is $E = X n_2 /n$. We note that O, being a count, is always a whole number whereas E need not be so. It is usually recorded correct to one or two decimals, depending on the magnitudes of the observed counts, with larger counts requiring less accuracy in E.

It is not necessary to calculate all the expected frequencies by this formula. Since the column totals are fixed (being the sample sizes $n_1, \ldots, n_k$), the expected number of observations of type F can be obtained as the difference between the sample sizes and the expected number of observations of type S.

2) After obtaining E for each cell, we calculate the statistic

$$Y = \Sigma \frac{(O - E)^2}{E}$$ (12.10)

where the summation is taken over all the 2k cells. Clearly, if each observed frequency is identical with what is expected under H_0, $Y = 0$, while the farther the observations are from the counts expected under H_0, the larger is Y. It follows that the significant values of Y are in the right tail of its distribution under H_0.

3) If the total n of all the sample sizes is large (and not many of the expected frequencies E are very small), Y has approximately a Chi-square distribution with $k-1$ degrees of freedom. Therefore, for a level α test of H_0, the significant values of Y are given by

$$Y > \chi^2_{k-1}(\alpha).$$ (12.11)

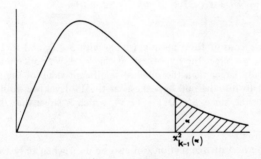

FIG. 12.5. The $100(1-\alpha)$th percentile of the Chi-square distribution with $k-1$ d.f.

Example 12.3. In a study of factors which may influence children aged between 10 and 12 1/2 years to start smoking, Bewley and Bland (1977) selected samples from four groups of school children in that age bracket and collected several items of pertinent information about each child. The groups were: heavy smokers, light smokers, experimental smokers and non-smokers. In these four populations, we take as the dichotomous variable the child's attitude towards the assertion that smoking is a health hazard, letting it be S if the child agrees with the assertion and F otherwise. We apply steps 1 to 3 above to test the hypothesis that the proportion of children who believe smoking to be a health hazard is the same in all four populations, using a 5% level of significance. The 2 x 4 table of *observed* frequencies, condensed from the authors' data, is the following:

	Heavy smokers	Light smokers	Experimental smokers	Non-smokers	Total
S	31	107	151	158	447
F	2	19	15	8	44
Total	33	126	166	166	491

Using Formula (12.9), we calculate the corresponding table of *expected* frequencies:

30.04	114.71	151.12	151.12
2.96	11.29	14.88	14.88

Applying Formula (12.10), we obtain the value of the test statistic:

$$Y = .03 + 1.87 + 0 + .31 + .31 + 5.27 + 0 + 3.18$$
$$= 10.97.$$

Since $k = 4$, we consult the Chi-square table with 3 d.f., and find $\chi_3^2 (.05) = 7.81$. Since $Y > 7.81$, we reject the hypothesis at this level. We notice that the calculated Y is not dramatically larger than the smallest significant value of the statistic. In fact, if we had decided to test the null hypothesis at the 1% level, we would have arrived at a different conclusion, since $\chi_3^2 (.01) = 11.34$, which is larger than the calculated value of Y.

Note (1). The method of this section can also be used when only two populations are compared. In fact, the statistic Y of Formula (12.10) can be shown to reduce to the *uncorrected* statistic Y of Formula (12.6) when k is 2. We have dealt with the case $k = 2$ separately for several reasons, of which we mention that Formula (12.10) calls for more calculations than the formulas of Section 12.1, that no correction for continuity is available for Formula (12.10), and that in the case of two samples it is limited to testing against a two-sided alternative.

Note (2). The test described in this section is applicable when no particular alternative is specified. If the populations can be meaningfully ordered, it is possible to test H_0 against an alternative of trend, such as $H_A : p_1 \leqslant p_2 \leqslant ... \leqslant p_k$. A test of the hypothesis of no trend against the alternative H_A, due to Armitage (1955), is described in — for instance — Brown and Hollander (1977), Armitage (1971), and Snedecor and Cochran (1967).

Note (3). A 2 x k table is not always the result of observations on k independent samples of fixed sizes, as in the model of this section. A *single* sample may be cross-classified according to two criteria, one of which has 2 categories and the other k categories, and the classification summarized in a 2 x k table of frequencies. The main question of inte-rest in such a sample is whether the row and column classifications are independent, and a test of the hypothesis of independence will be given in the next chapter without limiting the number of rows to 2. It will be seen that the mechanics of that test are identical with those of the test given in this section, and therefore the same computer programs can be used to calculate the test statistic in the two problems. The relevant program in Chapter 18 is Program CHIS3.

REFERENCES

Armitage, P. (1955). Tests for linear trends in proportions and frequencies. Biometrics, journal of The Biometric Society, *11*, 375-386.

Armitage, P. (1971). *Statistical Methods in Medical Research.* Blackwell Scientific Publi-cations, Oxford, England.

Barnett, V.D. (1969). Simultaneous pairwise linear structural relationships. Biometrics, journal of The Biometric Society, *25*, 129-142.

Bewley, B.R. and Bland, J.M. (1977). Academic performance and social factors related to cigarette smoking by school-children. Br. J. prev. soc. Med. *31*, 18-24.

Brown, B.W. and Hollander, M. (1977). *Statistics: A Biomedical Introduction.* Wiley, New York.

Cochran, W.G. (1950). The comparison of percentages in matched samples. Biometrika *37*, 256-266.

Lamoureux, G., Giard, N., Jolicoeur, R., Toughlian, V., and Desrosiers, M. (1976). Immu-nological features in multiple sclerosis. Br. med. J., Jan. 1976, 183-186.

Pearson, E.S. and Hartley, H.O. (editors) (1966). *Biometrika Tables for Statisticians*, vol. I, 3rd ed., Cambridge University Press, Cambridge, England.

Snedecor, G.W. and Cochran, W.G. (1967). *Statistical Methods*, 6th ed., Iowa State Uni-versity Press, Ames, Iowa, U.S.A.

Sokal, R.R. and Rohlf, F.J. (1969). *Biometry.* Freeman and Co., San Francisco, U.S.A.

CHAPTER 13
Association Between Two
Qualitative Variables

13.1. CONTINGENCY TABLES

One is often interested in the association between two qualitative variables observed on the same subject. Classic examples of such pairs of variables are the color of eyes and color of hair in human subjects, or the number of children in a family and the mother's level of education. In both of these examples, a certain amount of association is taken for granted without the benefit of statistical analysis, but it is quite possible that the association is a lot stronger in the first example than in the second, and therefore the degree of association may also be of interest.

In many investigations, the main question is whether the two variables are associated at all. If they are not associated, the probability of observing a certain category of one variable (say blue eyes) is not affected by observing any category of the other (say light hair or dark hair) in the same person. This means that, if the two variables are not associated, their categories are events which are independent of each other. In this case, the variables themselves are called *independent*.

Suppose that a sample of size n has been taken from a bivariate categorical population, and that the first variable is observed to fall into r different categories while the second is observed to fall into c different categories. Thus every observation consists of two statements, each statement specifying the category in which the corresponding variable falls. Since there are rc combinations of categories, the observations can be summarized in a table of rc frequencies arranged in r rows and c columns, as in the following r x c table, where we denote the frequency observed simultaneously in the ith row category and jth column category by O_{ij} ($i = 1, \ldots, r; j = 1, \ldots, c$).

Such a table of frequencies is known as a *contingency table*. The sum of all the entries in the table is the sample size n.

To test the independence (or lack of association) of the two variables that constitute the two criteria of classification, we follow a procedure similar to the one used to test the equality of k proportions in Section 12.3. In this case, the hypothesis tested is

H_0: the two variables are independent

Categories of the second variable

		1	2	.	.	.	c
Categories	1	O_{11}	O_{12} ·		·	·	O_{1c}
of the first	2	O_{21}	O_{22} ·		·	·	O_{2c}
variable							
	·	·					
	·	·					
	·	·					
	r	O_{r1}	O_{r2} ·		·	·	O_{rc}

and the procedure, in the notation of this chapter, is as follows:

1) Calculate the totals of all r rows; as a check, their sum must be n. Similarly, calculate the totals of all c columns and check that their sum is n.

2) For each cell, calculate the frequency that would be expected if, with the row and column totals as calculated in step 1, the row and column classifications are independent. For the cell in the ith row and jth column (which we refer to as the ij-th cell), this expected frequency is

$$E_{ij} = \text{(total of ith row) (total of jth column)}/n, \tag{13.1}$$

and this is not necessarily an integer.

It is easy to see why this formula gives the frequencies expected under independence. For, in the case of independence between the categories of the two variables, and with the given row and column totals, P(the observation falls in row i and column j)

$$= P(\text{it falls in row i}).P(\text{it falls in column j})$$

$$= \frac{total\ of\ ith\ row}{n} \cdot \frac{total\ of\ jth\ column}{n}$$

$$= p_{ij}, \text{ say .}$$

In a sample of size n, an observation either falls in the ij-th cell (the special category of a binomial variable) or it does not, and the expected number of observations of this type is $n\,p_{ij}$, as in Formula (13.1).

Although every E_{ij} must be calculated, it is not necessary to use Formula (13.1) for all of them, except as an additional check on the calculations. Any entry in the last row or last column or both can be obtained as the difference between the row (or column) total and the sum of the other entries in the same row (or column). Thus only $(r-1)\,(c-1)$ of the E_{ij} have to be calculated by this formula.

3) After obtaining the r x c table of the E_{ij} frequencies, calculate the statistic

$$Y = \Sigma_{i,j} \frac{(O_{ij} - E_{ij})^2}{E_{ij}} , \qquad (13.2)$$

where the sum is taken over all the rc cells. This statistic is zero if all the observed frequencies coincide with those expected under the hypothesis of independence. Since a certain amount of discrepancy between observed and expected frequencies may be due to random fluctuations, Y can also take positive values when the two variables are independent. When the discrepancy is too wide to be attributed to chance alone, Y is very large and the hypothesis of independence is rejected.

4) Under H_0 , the statistic Y has approximately a Chi-square distribution with $(r-1)(c-1)$ degrees of freedom, which is the same as the number of expected frequencies calculated without a restriction on their total. (The approximation is fairly good when n is large and not many E_{ij} very small). Therefore, at level α, the significant values of Y are given by

$$Y > \chi^2_{(r-1)(c-1)}(\alpha) . \qquad (13.3)$$

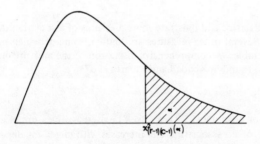

FIG. 13.1.   The $100(1-\alpha)$ th   percentile of the Chi-square distribution with $(r-1)$ $(c-1)$ d.f.

The value of Y for a given contigency table can also be obtained by   means   of Program CHIS3 of Chapter 18.

Example 13.1.   In a study of the use of minor tranquilizers in a non-institutionalized adult population, Uhlenhuth *et al* (1978) classified a sample of 735 respondents by criteria of age, sex, race, marital status, level of drug use, etc. To illustrate the methods of this section, we reproduce a cross-classification of 144 responses of drug users by marital status and level of drug use in Table 13.1 and test the hypothesis that, among users of prescription minor tranquilizers in that community, marital status and level of drug use are independent. Next to each observed frequency in the table, we have entered the expected frequency calculated as in step 2 above. Formula (13.2) was then used to calculate Y = 2.23. Since $\chi^2_4(.05) = 9.49$, an application of (13.3) leads us to accept the hypothesis tested at the 5% level.

Table 13.1.   Observed and expected frequencies   (O : E) in Example 13.1.

		Level of Use		
		Low	Medium	High
	Married	30 : 32.89	15 : 12.89	19 : 18.22
Marital status	Single	17 : 14.90	6 : 5.84	6 : 8.26
	Other	27 : 26.21	8 : 10.27	16 : 14.52

Source :   Uhlenhuth *et al.* Copyright 1978, American Medical Association.

13.2.   MEASURES OF ASSOCIATION

In this section we define and illustrate some measures of association that are applicable to any r x c table. Several other measures are known, some of which have been devised for special types of tables. A comprehensive discussion of the measurement of association in r x c tables can be found in Kendall and Stuart (1967).

a. The statistic Y of Formula (13.2) can itself be used as a measure of association, since it is zero in the case of no association and increases with increasing departure from independence. It has the disadvantage of having in general no upper limit for its value. However, since it is always calculated for the test of independence anyway, a closer look at it may provide more information at no extra cost.

We recall that, for a Chi-square variable with r degrees of freedom, the population mean (also known as the expected value) is r. Therefore, if the hypothesis of independence is true and the sample size is sufficiently large for Y to be considered as a Chi-square variable, the expected value of Y is $(r-1)(c-1)$. Dividing the calculated Y by its expected value under H_0 yields a quick measure of association which can be useful in comparing tables with different degrees of freedom.

Example 13.2.   To illustrate the use of Y as a measure of association, we use some of the data reported by Bewley and Bland (1977), and referred to in Example 12.3, concerning the smoking habits of schoolchildren. The numerical entries in the following tables are observed frequencies.

Table 13.2 Smoking habits of teenage boys and fathers

		Boys			
		Heavy smokers	Light smokers	Experimental smokers	Non-smokers
Fathers :	Smokers	25	65	89	71
	Non-smokers	6	21	34	52

Source : Bewley and Brand (1977)

Table 13.3 Smoking habits of teenage boys and brothers

		Boys			
		Heavy smokers	Light smokers	Experimental smokers	Non-smokers
Brothers :	None	5	19	43	43
	No smokers	12	39	55	70
	One smoker or more	14	28	25	9

Source : Bewley and Bland (1977)

Applying the method of Section 13.1, we calculated Y for the data in the two tables and obtained

Table	Calculated Y	d.f.	Y/d.f.
13.2	11.63	3	3.88
13.3	33.98	6	5.66

Both values of Y are significant at the 1% level. However, while in Table 13.2 Y is about 4 times its expected value, in Table 13.3 the ratio is a good bit larger (about 5 2/3) and indicates a stronger association.

b. Pearson's coefficient of contingency, defined as

$$P = \left(\frac{Y}{n + Y} \right)^{1/2},$$
(13.4)

has the advantage over Y of being no less than zero and no more than 1. When the two variables are not associated, $Y = 0$ and hence $P = 0$. However, the maximum value that P can take, even in the case of the strongest association, is less than 1 and depends on the size of the table.

c. Cramér's coefficient

$$C = \left(\frac{Y}{n \min (r-1, c-1)} \right)^{1/2}.$$

(13.5)

This coefficient is also between 0 and 1 but, unlike P, it is equal to 1 in the extreme case of perfect dependence between the variables, where only one category of one variable is possible with a given category of the other.

Example 13.3. From the data of Example 13.2, we calculated the coefficients P and C as follows:–

Table	Y	P	C
13.2	11.63	.18	.18
13.3	33.98	.29	.22

Both measures, like the ratio of Y to its expected value, show a stronger association in the second of the two tables.

REFERENCES

Kendall, M.G. and Stuart, A. (1967). *The Advanced Theory of Statistics.* vol II, 2nd ed. Charles Griffin and Co., London.

Uhlenhuth, E.E., Balter, M.B., and Lipman, R.S. (1978). Minor tranquilizers: Clinical correlates of use in an urban population. Archs gen. Psychiat. *35*, 650-655.

Bewley, B.R. and Bland, J.M. (1977). Academic performance and social factors related to cigarette smoking by schoolchildren. Br. J. Prev. soc. Med. *31*, 18-24.

CHAPTER 14
Association Between Two Numerical Variables

14.1. REGRESSION AND THE METHOD OF LEAST SQUARES

In this chapter, we consider numerical data of the bivariate type. Two variables, X and Y, are observed simultaneously and their values, in whatever units are convenient for each, are recorded as an ordered pair of numbers (x,y). The purpose is to study the relationship, if any, between the two variables, using a sample of the ordered pairs (x,y). The first step in such a study usually consists of drawing the *scatter diagram* of the data, which is a plot of the n points in the Cartesian plane corresponding to the n ordered pairs of the sample (as was described in Section 3.4 c). In the scatter diagram, association is indicated by a clustering of the points around a line or a curve suggesting that, although corresponding to a given X the Y values may fluctuate above and below a certain average, this *average* value of Y depends on the given value of X, and a change in X produces a corresponding change in the Y average. This dependence of the average values of Y on the other variable is known as the *regression of Y on X*, and the equation of the line or curve that summarizes this dependence for all values of X is known as the *regression function*. The statistical analysis of regression has many different uses, some of which are illustrated in the following examples.

Example 14.1. The main object in this example was to find out *if an association could be assumed to exist* between the two variables. Hiller *et al* (1977), using data from two large U.S. sources, recorded the prevalence of cataract and the corresponding amount of sunlight in their geographical location for subjects of several age groups. Their variables were

X = annual sunlight (in 100 hours)

Y = ratio of cataract to control cases.

For a number of different age groups,   they studied the values of Y at different levels of X and found that, for persons 65 years or older, Y showed an overall increase corresponding to an increase in X. No such association was apparent in other age groups, and the findings were not considered conclusive.

Example 14.2.   While accepting it as known that mortality rates from coronary heart disease increase with age, Heller and Jacobs (1978) investigated the *speed with which this increase occurs* before and after the menopause in the two sexes. Their variables were

X = age (in years)

Y = death rate (per 1000 pop./year).

They found that the rate at which the average value of Y increased with X was considerably lower in men for whom X > 50.

Example 14.3.   Henry and Altmann (1978) found that hypoproteinaemic oedema pits and recovers at a different rate from other types of oedema. For a group of oedematous patients, they observed the variables

X = pit recovery time (in seconds)

Y = serum albumin (in g/1)

and found in their sample a clear regression of Y on X. As a result, they suggested that pitting time X, which is an easily observed physical phenomenon, can be used in *predicting the corresponding value of Y*, and hence in the diagnosis of hypoproteinaemic oedema.

Example 14.4.   A sample of 28 systolic blood pressure determinations from a group of Lebanese women employees over 35 years old (Abou-Daoud, 1979) had a mean equal to 123.6 mm and a standard deviation equal to 19.14 mm. Since this somewhat large variability in blood pressure may be due, at least in part, to the differences in the ages of the employees, we considered the variables

X = age (in years)

Y = systolic blood pressure (in mm of Hg)

and investigated the regression of Y on X. By methods which will be described in the next section, we *eliminated the effect of X on the variation in Y* and calculated the residual standard deviation in the latter. This we found to be 17.72 mm, so that eliminating the effect of X did not appreciably reduce the variation in Y.

All of the above examples involved the regression of one variable on another, yet the purpose of the investigation in each case was of a completely different nature, and the conclusions dealt with different aspects of the association between the variables.

Some information about the association between two numerical variables can always be obtained from an inspection of the sample scatter diagram. Consider, for example, the six scatter diagrams in Figure 14.1. The plots in (a) and (d) suggest that in both cases Y decreases on the average as X inscreases, and that the regression of Y on X in the population very likely follows a straight line with a negative slope; the two plots differ, however, in the closeness of the points to the line describing their trend, with the plot in (d) showing a stronger association between X and Y than the one in (a). An association between the variables is also apparent in (b) and in (e), but the regression functions in these two cases do not appear to be linear, since the points in each diagram can be seen to fall along a curve rather than a straight line. The scatter diagrams (c) and (f) reveal no regression of Y on X, since the average height of the points above the X axis in each case seems to be the same for all values of X.

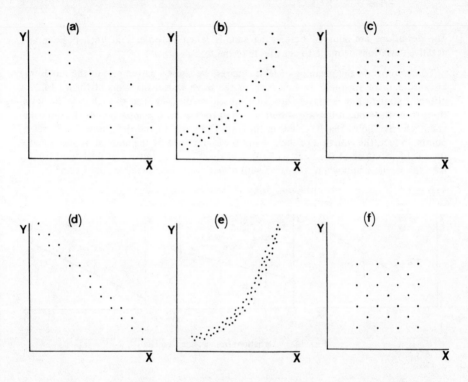

FIG. 14.1. Some examples of scatter diagrams

Whatever type of regression function is suggested by the scatter diagram, the next step in the analysis is to find its equation from the sample data. This involves finding the constants of the equation, like the constants a and b in the equation of the straight line $Y = a + bX$, or the constants a, b and c in the equation of the parabola $Y = a + bX + cX^2$, etc. For the case of the straight line, a and b can be calculated from the sample data by formulas which will be given in the next section. The formulas were derived by a method known as the method of *least squares*, which can in principle be used to derive the constants for other and more complicated equations. It is based on the principle that the better a curve (or line) describes a trend in the scatter diagram the less is the total deviation of the plotted points from it, each deviation being squared before being added to the total. By the "deviation" of a point (x_i, y_i) from the curve is meant its *vertical* deviation or, more precisely, the difference between the ordinate y_i of the point and the ordinate of a point on the curve having the same abscissa x_i. It is the sum of the squares of such deviations over the whole sample that is minimized by this method, so that, for a curve with equation $Y = f(X)$, the quantity that is minimized is

$$\sum_{i=1}^{n} [y_i - f(x_i)]^2 \ .$$

The deviations are squared before the sum is taken in order that both positive and negative deviations be made to contribute to the total.

To demonstrate the meaning of least squares, we show a partial plot of the Age-Blood Pressure data of Example 14.4 in each of the three scatter diagrams of Figure 14.2. A different straight line is drawn through each scatter diagram, and in each case the deviations from the straight line are also indicated in the figure. A comparison of the three diagrams clearly shows that the line in (c) is the "closest" of the three lines to the set of points. In fact, the equation of the line in (c) was obtained by the method of least squares (using the formulas of the next section), and therefore the squares of deviations from it have the smallest sum when compared with deviations from *any other* straight line.

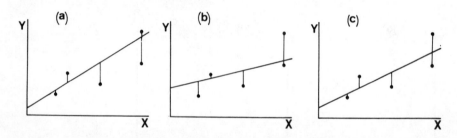

FIG. 14.2.   Deviations from a regression line

14.2.   LINEAR REGRESSION

14.2 a.   Population Regression Line

When the regression of Y on X is linear, the population values of X and Y are such that when X takes a specific value x, the corresponding average value of Y is the linear function

$$\mu(x) = \alpha + \beta\, x, \tag{14.1}$$

which is also known as the equation of the *population regression line*. The constants α and β are, respectively, the intercept and slope of this line. Of the two, α is simply the average value of Y corresponding to $X = 0$, which has a practical meaning only if zero is one of the possible values of X. The other parameter, β, known as the *population regression coefficient,* carries more information about the relationship between the two variables. Being the slope of the regression line, it is positive if $\mu(x)$ increases with x, negative if $\mu(x)$ decreases with x, and zero if $\mu(x)$ is not affected by x. More precisely, β is the change in $\mu(x)$ when x is increased by 1 unit; in the absence of regression, β is zero.

14.2 b. Sample Regression Line

The population parameters, α and β, are usually unknown, and their estimates are obtained from the sample of ordered pairs (x, y). Denote the sum of squares of deviations of the sample points from the line (14.1) by S, so that $S = \Sigma |(y_i - \alpha - \beta x_i)^2$. To find the values of the parameters α and β that minimize S, we differentiate it with respect to α and β, equate the derivatives to zero, and solve the resulting equations. The solutions are the *least squares* estimates of α and β which are given below.

We shall use the notation

$$S(x,y) = \Sigma x_i y_i - (\Sigma x_i)(\Sigma y_i)/n$$
$$S(x,x) = \Sigma x_i^2 - (\Sigma x_i)^2/n \qquad\qquad (14.2)$$
$$S(y,y) = \Sigma y_i^2 - (\Sigma y_i)^2/n,$$

which will also be found convenient elsewhere in this chapter. In this notation, the least squares estimates of α and β are:

$$\hat{\beta} = b = S(x,y)/S(x,x) \qquad\qquad (14.3)$$

$$\hat{\alpha} = a = \overline{y} - b\overline{x},$$

where $\overline{x} = \Sigma x_i/n$ and $\overline{y} = \Sigma y_i/n$. Replacing α and β in the population regression equation by their estimates, we obtain the equation of the *sample regression line*

$$\hat{\mu}(x) = a + bx \qquad\qquad (14.4)$$

which gives the estimated average value of Y corresponding to a specified x. This equation can also be obtained by means of Program REGS1 of Chapter 18.

14.2 c. Semi-Log and Log-Log Graphs

In addition to a wide variety of problems in which the scatter diagram shows the relation between the variables to be of the linear type, there are cases where the relation can be made linear by applying an appropriate transformation to one or both of the variables. The transformed data can then be analyzed by the methods of linear regression.

Two such transformations, the semi-log and the log-log transformations, were discussed and illustrated in Chapter 3 (Section 3.4). The first is used if the relation between X and Y can be roughly described by the equation $Y = cd^X$, where c and $d > 0$ are constants. Taking the logarithm of Y (to the base 10) and making it the new variable Y′, we get $Y' = c' + d'X$, which is a straight line relation between Y′ and the original variable X. The second transformation is used if the relation in the original data can be roughly described by the equation $Y = cX^d$. In this case, transforming both X and Y by taking their logarithms, we obtain the linear relation $Y' = c' + dX'$ between the transformed variables. The equations of the sample regression lines in the transformed variables can be obtained directly by means of Program REGS2 of Chapter 18.

Example 14.5. The length X (in cm) and the weight Y (in gm) for 55 specimens of *Pagellus acarne** are plotted in the scatter diagram (a) of Figure 14.3. Since the pattern of points in the scatter diagram suggests that a semi-logarithmic transformation might be appropriate, we replaced each observed y_i by log y_i and plotted the ordered pairs $(x_i, \log y_i)$ as the scatter diagram (b) of Figure 14.3. For the transformed data the regression of log Y on X appears to be linear, and the least squares regression line drawn in the figure has the equation

$$\hat{\mu}(x) = -1.08 + .24x.$$

This equation was found by calculating a and b as in Formulas (14.3), with log y being used in the place of y, and substituting in (14.4).

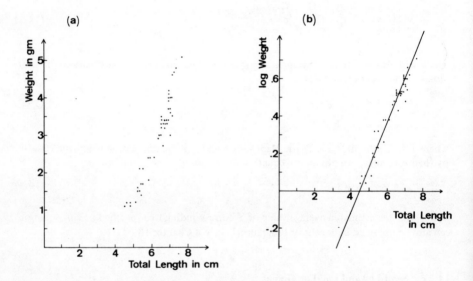

FIG. 14.3. Use of the semi-log transformation (Example 14.5)

In interpreting this result, we must keep in mind that it is the logarithm of Y that increases, on the average, at the constant rate of .24 grams per centimeter increase in X. In fact, starting with any two points on the regression line, if X is increased by one unit, log Y is increased by .24 of a unit, and hence Y is *multiplied by a factor of* $10^{.24} = 1.74$.

---

* Data source: Biology Department, American University of Beirut.

14.2d. Segmented Regression Lines

Some scatter diagrams may show a changing pattern of regression that can best be described by a sequence of connected regression lines with different slopes. The change in slope usually occurs at values of X which are in some way critical for the behavior of Y, as at points c and d of Figure 14.4. The equation of each of the line segments is found by the least squares Formulas (14.3) and (14.4) applied to a portion of the sample data, with an overlap in the data sets used for any two adjacent line segments. In Figure 14.4, for instance, each of the sets of encircled points is used twice: once as belonging to a portion of the scatter diagram immediately on its left, and once as belonging to a portion on its right.

Example 14.6. Sweatman and Koussa (1968) observed the respiration of engorged female ticks on the day of peak metabolic rate and found a temperature "break point" of 30°C in the regression of the metabolic rate on temperature, with an increasing rate for temperatures below 30°C and a decreasing rate above it. The scatter diagram for their data and the fitted regression line segments are shown in Figure 14.5.

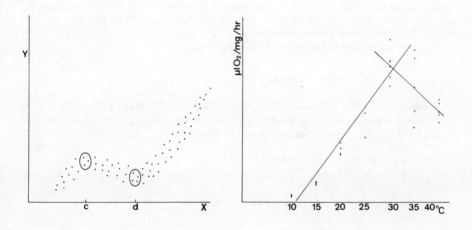

FIG. 14.4. Linear regression in segments

FIG. 14.5. Linear regression for data of Example 14.6.

14.2 e. Normality Assumption

If the purpose of the analysis is only to estimate the regression of Y on X, then Equations (14.3) and (14.4) are sufficient. For stages in the analysis beyond this descriptive stage, like testing hypotheses about the parameters or using the regression line for making probability statements about predictions, some assumptions about the distribution of Y

are needed in addition to the regression function (14.1). The usual assumptions in the linear regression model are the following:
For each fixed value x of the variable X,

(i) Y has a normal distribution,
(ii) the mean of Y is $\alpha + \beta x$, where α and β are constants, and   (14.5)
(iii) the standard deviation of Y is σ, the same for all x.

We note that σ is a measure of the fluctuations of Y about its mean and hence its fluctuations above and below the regression line. Therefore, no matter what effect X may have on the average of Y, whether the regression line is rising or falling, and whether its slope is large or small, σ is not affected and reflects only the random variations in Y.

An unbiased estimate of the square of σ is the mean square

$$s^2 = \frac{\Sigma (y_i - \hat{\mu}(x_i))^2}{n - 2}$$ (14.6)

where $\hat{\mu}(x_i)$ is given in (14.4), and the summation is over the n elements of the sample. Thus the numerator of this estimate is the minimized sum of squared deviations. When written in the from $\Sigma(y_i - a - bx_i)^2$, this sum is seen to be the sum of n different squares with two restrictions imposed on them, the restrictions being a and b as defined in Equations (14.3). Hence its degrees of freedom are n−2.
A simpler computational form for s^2 is the following:

$$s^2 = (\Sigma y_i^2 - a \, \Sigma y_i - b \, \Sigma x_i y_i)/(n-2) \, .$$ (14.7)

Example 14.7.   The data shown in the scatter diagrams of Figure 14.2 consisted of the following ordered pairs (x,y) where the variable X represents age (in years) and the variable Y the systolic blood pressure (in mm of mercury)

    x :   40   48   58   58   37
    y :   120   115   140   125   110

The reader can easily verify the following calculations:

    $\Sigma x = 241$ $\Sigma y = 610$ $n = 5$
    $\Sigma x^2 = 12001$ $\Sigma y^2 = 74950$ $\Sigma xy = 29760$.

From (14.3) we get a = 77.17 and b = .93. Therefore the regression line of this small sample has the equation $\hat{\mu}(x) = 77.17 + .93x$. This line is drawn in Figure 14.2 (c). To estimate the standard deviation of Y about the regression line, we use Formula (14.7) and obtain

$$s^2 = [74950 - (17.17)(610) - (.93)(29760)]/3$$
$$= 65.69,$$
therefore s = 8.10.

Note: In the above presentation of the linear regression model, the roles played by the two variables have been quite different. In general, if one of the two variables is such that its values can be controlled in the experiment (like time, dosage level, food intake, etc.), then this variable is taken as X and called the *predictor variable,* while Y (*the criterion variable*) is the one whose values are observed in the experiment. The distinction is not always so clear-cut, for in some investigations both variables are experimentally observed, and the regression of either one or the other or both may be of interest. Using the methods of this section, and by an appropriate labelling of the variables, the regression of either one on the other can be estimated. In some cases, one may wish to obtain equations of *two* regression lines: the line of regression of Y on X with which we have been dealing, and the line of regression of X on Y. The formulas for arriving at the equation of the latter can be obtained from those of the former by simply interchanging X and Y. When the two regression lines are drawn on the same scatter diagram, they should intersect at the point $(\bar{x}, \bar{y})$. This can be used as a check on the calculations.

14.3. INFERENCE ABOUT A REGRESSION LINE

Some commonly used inference procedures in linear regression problems will be described in this section. The procedures will be illustrated numerically at the end of the section in Example 14.8.

In these inference methods, we consider X as a *controlled variable* in the sense that it assumes fixed values preassigned by the experimenter, while Y is allowed to vary in accordance with the set of assumptions (14.5). When X must also be considered as subject to random variations, so that a different sample may very well produce a different set of X values, we may still use the same methods, taking the observed values of X as though they were fixed in advance and analyzing the Y values under that condition.

14.3 a. Inference concerning the regression coefficient

We have already seen how β can be estimated by b from a given bivariate sample $(x_1, y_1), \ldots, (x_n, y_n)$. Keeping $x_1, \ldots, x_n$ fixed, and taking into account all the possible values of Y in the population, we now consider the sample regression coefficient as a variable, say B, whose value calculated from a given sample is b, and which is defined as

$$B = \frac{\Sigma_i x_i Y_i - (\Sigma x_i)(\Sigma Y_i)/n}{S(x,x)}$$

If the assumptions (14.5) are satisfied, B is a normal variable with mean equal to β and standard error equal to $\sigma/\sqrt{S(x,x)}$. Replacing σ by its estimate s from Formula (14.7), we get the estimated standard error of B as $s/\sqrt{S(x,x)}$, and hence the variable

$$T = \frac{B - \beta}{s/\sqrt{S(x,x)}}$$

has a t-distribution with n−2 degrees of freedom.

To test the hypothesis

$$H_0 : \ \beta = \beta_0$$

at significance level α, we calculate the value of the statistic T when H_0 is true as

$$T_0 = \frac{b - \beta_0}{s / \sqrt{S(x,x)}} \tag{14.8}$$

using Formulas (14.2), (14.3) and (14.7), and reject H_0

against right-sided alternatives if $T_0 > t_{n-2}(\alpha)$,

against left-sided alternatives if $T_0 < - t_{n-2}(\alpha)$,

against two-sided alternatives if $|T_0| > t_{n-2}(\alpha/2)$.

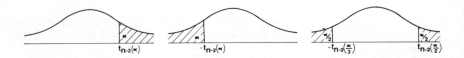

FIG. 14.6. Percentiles of the t−distribution with n−2 d.f..

When the hypothesis gives β_0 as zero, it becomes the hypothesis of no regression, and the test is meant to find out whether or not X can be assumed to have any effect on the average value of Y.

Using the distribution of the variable T, one can also construct a confidence interval for β. At a confidence level of $1-\alpha$, the limits of the interval are

$$b \pm t_{n-2}(\alpha/2).s \sqrt{S(x,x)}. \tag{14.9}$$

14.3 b.   Analysis of variance for regression

The calculations for testing the hypothesis $H_0 : \beta = 0$ can also be displayed in an analysis of variance table. In such a table, the total variation in Y is divided into its two main sources: regression on X, and deviation from regression (or randomness). The sum of squares due to each of the sources, and the corresponding mean squares, are shown in Table 14.1.

The quantities S(x,y), S(xx) and S(y,y) were defined in (14.2), and the mean square for deviation from regression is the estimate of σ^2 defined in (14.6). The variance ratio $b^2 S(x,x)/s^2$, which is the value of an F variable with 1 and n−2 degrees of freedom if H_0 is true, is precisely the square of T_0 of (14.8), with β_0 replaced by zero, and can therefore be used to test the hypothesis of no regression. This is no coincidence, since an F variable with 1 degree of freedom in its numerator is the square of a t-variable having the same degrees of freedom as in its denominator. We observe that the F test based on the analysis of variance can replace the t-test of no regression only when the alternatives are two-sided.

Table 14.1 Analysis of variance for linear regression

Source of variation	Sum of squares	Degrees of freedom	Mean square
Regression	$(S(x,y))^2/S(x,x)$	1	$b^2 S(x,x)$
Deviation from regression	$\Sigma (y_i - \hat{\mu}(x_i))^2$	$n-2$	s^2
Total	$S(y,y)$	$n-1$	

14.3 c. Inference concerning the height of the regression line

Corresponding to any given value of X, say x_0, μ is estimated by the variable

$$\hat{\mu}(x_0) = A + Bx_0,$$

where $A = \overline{Y} - B\overline{x}$ and B is as defined in section **14.3 a** above. If the assumptions (14.5) are satisfied, $\hat{\mu}(x_0)$ is a normally distributed variable, with mean equal to $\mu(x_0)$, and standard error equal to

$$s\sqrt{\frac{1}{n} + \frac{(x_0 - \overline{x})^2}{S(x,x)}},$$

with $S(x,x)$ as given in (14.2). It follows that the variable

$$T = \frac{(A + Bx_0) - \mu(x_0)}{s\sqrt{\frac{1}{n} + \frac{(x_0 - \overline{x})^2}{S(x,x)}}},$$

where s is the estimate of σ given in (14.6) and (14.7), has a t-distribution with $n-2$ degrees of freedom. Therefore, a $1-\alpha$ confidence interval for μ at $X = x_0$, based on the variable T, is given by

$$(a + bx_0) \pm t_{n-2}(\alpha/2).s\sqrt{\frac{1}{n} + \frac{(x_0 - \overline{x})^2}{S(x,x)}}, \tag{14.10}$$

where a and b were defined in (14.3) and $t_{n-2}(\alpha/2)$ is sketched in Figure 14.6.

Graphically, (14.10) can be marked on the scatter diagram as a vertical interval above $X = x_0$. It is obtained in such a way that one can be fairly confident (confident at level $1-\alpha$) that the population regression line passes through the interval.

If several such intervals are calculated, each for a different value of X but at the same confidence level, they can be used to draw a *confidence band* for the population regression line. The upper boundary of this band consists of a curve drawn through the upper limits of the confidence intervals, and the lower boundary is drawn through their lower limits. The probability that the band contains the population regression line within its boundaries is then the confidence level $1-\alpha$. A confidence band for the data of Example 14.8 is shown in Figure 14.7.

14.3 d. Prediction of a Y value

Occasionally, one is interested in an individual value of Y corresponding to a given x, rather than in the average $\mu(x)$. Suppose that a regression line has been determined from a sample of size n, and that we wish to predict the value of Y corresponding to x_0 in an additional observation, where x_0 is somewhere in the range of the observed values of X. In the absence of more information, the best that we can do by way of prediction is to estimate the *average* Y at x_0 and use it as the predicted value. This, however, involves a larger error than estimating μ at x_0, and the larger error is reflected in a wider confidence interval. The confidence interval for the predicted value $Y(x_0)$ at level $1-\alpha$ is given by the limits

$$(a + bx_0) \pm t_{n-2}(\alpha/2). \sqrt{1 + \frac{1}{n} + \frac{(x_0 - \bar{x})^2}{S(x,x)}}. \tag{14.11}$$

Comparing this interval with the interval (14.10), we see that it is centered at the same point (namely $\hat{\mu}(x_0)$) but is considerably wider.

Since this method of prediction utilizes the estimates derived from the sample, it is valid only for a choice of x_0 within the range of observations. Extrapolation outside the sample range may lead to predictions that are grossly in error.

Example 14.8. To illustrate the calculations, we use Harakeh's (1978) data on the weight X (in grams) and mercury content Y (in $\mu g/kg$ weight) of fish caught off the Lebanese coast in 1977. Routine calculations on the data, which appears in Table 3.20 of Chapter 3, gave the following results:

$$\Sigma x_i \quad 952.9 \qquad \Sigma y_i = 1035 \qquad n = 21$$

$$\Sigma x_i^2 = 48034.37 \qquad \Sigma y_i^2 = 63931 \qquad \Sigma x_i y_i = 53121.0$$

Hence, by Formulas (14.2),

$$S(x,x) = 4795.40 \qquad S(y,y) = 12920.29 \qquad S(x,y) = 6156.64$$

and, by Formulas (14.3),

$$b = 1.2839 \quad \text{and} \quad a = -8.9728 .$$

This degree of accuracy in the estimates is needed for calculating s^2 but is otherwise not necessary. Substituting a and b in (14.4), we get the equation of the sample regression line,

$$\hat{\mu}(x) = -8.97 + 1.28x, \tag{14.12}$$

and, by (14.7), the estimated standard deviation from regression is

$$s = 16.25.$$

(a) To test the hypothesis $H_0 : \beta = 0$, against the alternative $H_R : \beta > 0,$ at the 5% level, we use (14.8) to calculate

$$T_0 = \frac{1.28 - 0}{16.25 / \sqrt{4795.40}} = 5.45.$$

This is larger than $t_{19}(.05) = 1.73$, and we therefore reject H_0 .

To obtain a 95% confidence interval for β, we look up the percentile $t_{19}(.025) = 2.093$ and use (14.9) to calculate the limits

$$1.28 \pm (2.093)(16.25) / \sqrt{4795.4}$$
$$\text{or} \quad (0.79, 1.77).$$

(b) We now test the hypothesis $H_0 : \beta = 0$ against a two-sided alternative at the 5% level, using the F ratio calculated from the analysis of variance table. In the notation of Table 14.1, the total and regression sums of squares are, respectively, 12920.29 and $(6156.64)^2 / 4795.40 = 7904.29$. The deviation sum of squares is obtained as their difference , and the other entries easily follow, resulting in the table:

Source	Sum of squares	d.f.	Mean square
Regression	7904.29	1	7904.29
Deviation	5016.00	19	264.00
Total	12920.29	20	

The ratio of the mean squares is 29.94, which is significant at the 5% level since it is larger than $F_{1,19}(.05) = 4.38$. H_0 is therefore rejected. Note that this result could have been anticipated from the fact that the 95% confidence interval for β that was found in the previous paragraph did not contain the number zero.

(c) To construct a 90% confidence band for the population regression line, we calculate intervals of the type given in (14.10) corresponding to $\alpha = 10\%$ and $x_0 = 20, 30, 40, 50, 60$ and 70. In this example, the interval (14.10) reduces to

$$-8.97 + 1.28x_0 \pm 28.11 \sqrt{\frac{1}{21} + \frac{(x_0 - 45.38)^2}{47950.40}}$$

and the limits are as tabulated below:

x_0	lower limit	upper limit
20	4.64	28.62
30	20.68	38.18
40	35.72	48.74
50	48.62	61.44
60	59.29	76.37
70	68.90	92.36

These limits are plotted on the scatter diagram in Figure 14.7, with the lower and upper limits connected to form a 90% confidence band for the population regression line. The sample regression line is also shown in the figure.

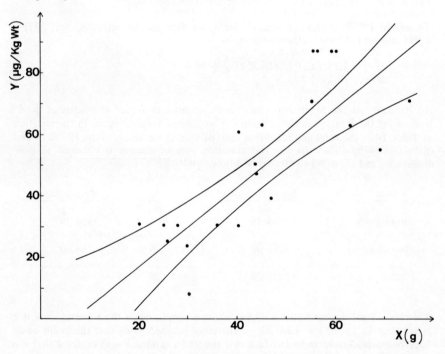

FIG. 14.7. Scatter diagram, sample regression line and 90% confidence band (Example 14.8)

(d) To predict the mercury concentration for an individual fish weighing exactly 50 grams, we use (14.11) to construct a 90% confidence interval for the predicted value which, by Equation (14.12), is $(1.28)(50) - 8.97 = 55.03$. The confidence interval is

$$55.03 \pm (1.73)(16.25)\sqrt{1 + \frac{1}{21} + \frac{21.34}{4795.4}}$$

or $(26.20, 83.86)$.

Statistics calculated in this example can also be obtained by Program REGS3 of Chapter 18.

14.4. LINEAR CORRELATION

Like linear regression, linear correlation is used to describe the relationship between two numerical variables whose scatter diagram shows a straight line tendency. However, while regression deals mainly with the position and direction of regression lines, correlation measures the closeness of the points to those lines. If all the points in a scatter diagram fall *on* a line, the association between X and Y is so complete that a value of one of the variables determines the corresponding value of the other exactly; on the other hand, the more dispersed the points are, the weaker is the association.

Unlike regression, correlation is a relationship in which the two variables play reciprocal roles, and rather than consider one of them as controlled and the other as varying at fixed levels of the first, we now assume that both X and Y are subject to random fluctuations from sample to sample.

Given a sample of ordered pairs $(x_1, y_1), \ldots, (x_n, y_n)$, a commonly used measure of the association between the two variables is the sample *coefficient of correlation*, usually denoted by r and, in the notation of Equations (14.2), defined as

$$r = \frac{S(x,y)}{\sqrt{S(x,x)S(y,y)}} \ . \tag{14.13}$$

r is also known as Pearson's product-moment coefficient of correlation.

This measure of association has the following properties that can be used in interpreting the value of r calculated from a particular sample:

(i)
$$r = b\sqrt{\frac{S(x,x)}{S(y,y)}} \ , \tag{14.14}$$

where b is the sample regression coefficient. This relation, which follows from the definition of r in (14.13) and the definition of b in (14.3), implies that r and b have the same sign. Therefore, a negative r means that Y decreases on the average as X increases, a positive r means that X and the average of Y increase together, and when $r = 0$ the sample coefficient of regression is also zero.

(ii)
$$0 \leqslant r^2 \leqslant 1 \ . \tag{14.15}$$

This can be seen from the partitioning of the total sum   of squares in the analysis of variance in Table 14.1. Since:
Regression sum of squares $\leqslant$ Total sum of squares,

$$(S(x,y))^2 / S(x,x) \leqslant S(y,y).$$

Dividing both sides of the inequality by the positive quantity $S(y,y)$, we get

$$(S(x,y))^2 / S(x,x)S(y,y) \leqslant 1,$$
$$\text{or} \qquad r^2 \qquad\qquad\qquad \leqslant 1,$$

so that the correlation coefficient r is a number between -1 and $+1$.

(iii) In the case of *maximum association*, when all the points in the scatter diagram fall on the same line,

$$r = \pm 1.$$

This can also be seen from Table 14.1, in which the Deviations sum of squares would be zero if all the points fell on the same line. Then the Regression sum of squares and the Total sum of squares would be equal, so that

$$(S(x,y))^2 / S(x,x) = S(y,y)$$

and $r^2 = 1$, hence $r = \pm 1$.

(iv) r^2 may be interpreted as *the fraction of the variation in Y that is due to variation in X*. If $r^2 = 1$, all the variation in Y is due to X, as in the previous paragraph. In general, and   again with   reference to   Table 14.1, since the Deviations   mean   square is $[S(y,y) - b^2 S(xx)]/ (n-2)$ and the Total mean square is $S(y,y)/(n-1)$, their ratio is

$$\frac{\text{Deviations mean square}}{\text{Total mean square}} = \frac{(n-1)}{(n-2)} \frac{[S(y,y) - b^2 S(x,x)]}{S(y,y)}$$

$$= \frac{(n-1)}{(n-2)} (1-r^2)$$

$$\cong 1-r^2.$$

Therefore $1-r^2$ is approximately the fraction of the total variation in Y that is due to randomness (or deviation from the line). It follows that its complement, r^2, is the fraction of the variation in Y that is due to the other factor, namely regression on X.

Example 14.9. From the data of Example 14.8, we calculate

$$r = \frac{6156.64}{\sqrt{(4795.4)(12920.29)}} = .78$$

and $r^2 = .61$.

We can therefore say that approximately 61% of the variation in the mercury concentration is due to variation in the weight of the fish. Note that the size of r itself is deceptively large, being much closer to 1 than to zero, and should not be interpreted as a relative measure of complete association between X and Y. In other words, a correlation of 78% is *not* 78% of the way to perfect association!

The value of r can also be read from the output of Program REGS1 in Chapter 18.

Note: Hand calculations of r can sometimes be considerably simplified if a constant were subtracted from each observation or if each observation were divided by a constant. Different transformations may be carried out on X and on Y. For instance, in Example 14.7, we can subtract 35 from each x and 110 from each y, with the resulting transformed sample

        x' :   5   13   23   23   2

        y' :   10   5   30   15   0

which reduces the necessary calculations. This is sometimes referred to as *coding* of the observations. Coding does not affect the value of r because, by its definition, r is independent of location or scale of measurement. This is not true of the regression coefficient b, and therefore little is gained from such a transformation if both b and r are to be calculated from the same set of data.

14.5. CURVILINEAR REGRESSION AND CORRELATION

Although linear regression provides an adequate model for most regression data, some scatter diagrams clearly suggest a *curvilinear* relationship (following a curve) that cannot be made linear by a simple transformation. An example of such a case is when the average Y is a function of the form

$$\mu(x) = a + bx + cx^2 \tag{14.16}$$

or, for that matter, any of the polynomial functions of degree higher than the first. As in the case of linear regression, two problems present themselves: (i) can one use the sample values to find the equation of the regression curve? and (ii) having found it, how can one measure the closeness of the observations to the curve?

(i) A regression function of a given type can usually be fitted to a set of data by the method of least squares, that is, by finding the constants of the function that minimize the sum of squared deviations from the regression curve. This is illustrated in Example 14.10 for a quadratic function of the form (14.16). More complicated functions, or functions involving a larger number of constants, would call for more tedious calculations than in the given example. However, when $\mu(x)$ is a sum of terms involving different functions of x (as it is in any polynomial), the methods of *multiple linear regression*, which is regression on several predictor variables, can be used, with each function of X playing the role of a different variable. We shall return to this topic in Section 14.8.

(ii) To measure the closeness of the points in the scatter diagram to the regression curve, we use a quantity known as the *correlation ratio*, denoted by η^2 (eta square), which is defined in a manner analogous to the measure r^2 in linear regression. For a given regression curve $\mu(x)$, consider the total variation in Y as made up of two components, variation along the curve $\mu(x)$, and random variation in the form of deviations from it. In other words, the Total sum of squares $S(y,y)$ can be divided into the Regression sum of squares and the Deviations sum of squares, the latter being $\Sigma(y_i - \hat{\mu}(x_i))^2$ where, as in the case of linear regression, $\hat{\mu}(x_i)$ is the value of the function $\mu(x)$ at the point x_i and with the constants in the function replaced by their least squares estimates.

In this context, the correlation ratio is defined as

$$\eta^2 = 1 - \frac{\text{Deviations sum of squares}}{\text{Total sum of squares}}$$

$$= 1 - \frac{\Sigma(y_i - \hat{\mu}(x_i))^2}{S(y,y)} . \tag{14.17}$$

Example 14.10. To illustrate these methods, we use the following observations on hydrolysis of urea (from an experiment by Gale and Eadie, as quoted by Bailey *et al* (1974)), in which X stands for time (in mins.) and Y for concentration of CO_2 (in percent). The plot of the observations in Figure 14.8 suggests that a regression function of the form

$$\mu(x) = a + bx + cx^2$$

might be appropriate. To find the least squares estimates of a, b and c, we take the sum of squared deviations of the points (x_i, y_i) from $\mu(x)$, which is

$$S = \sum_i (y_i - a - bx_i - cx_i^2)^2 ,$$

differentiate it with respect to each of a, b and c in turn, and equate each derivative to zero. The result is the following three equations in the three unknowns: a, b and c.

$$na + b\Sigma x_i + c\Sigma x_i^2 = \Sigma y_i$$

$$a\,\Sigma x_i + b\Sigma x_i^2 + c\Sigma x_i^3 = \Sigma x_i y_i$$

$$a\,\Sigma x_i^2 + b\Sigma x_i^3 + c\Sigma x_i^4 = \Sigma x_i y_i^2 .$$

Solving the three equations simultaneously, we get

$$a = -6.85$$

$$a = 8.15$$

$$c = 0.175$$

and therefore the parabola that best fits the data has the equation

$$\hat{\mu}(x) = -6.85 + 8.15x - .175x^2 .$$

This curve is also shown in Figure 14.8
The curve shows an exceptionally good fit for this data set, and this closeness of the points to it should be reflected in the value of the correlation ratio η^2. With such a small sample, it was easy to calculate the Deviations sum of squares directly by finding $\hat{\mu}(x_i)$, which is the height of the parabola, for each sample point (x_i,y_i), and adding the squares of $y_i - \hat{\mu}(x_i)$ over the 10 sample elements. These calculations gave the Deviations sum of squares as

$$\sum_i (y_i - \hat{\mu}(x_i))^2 = 12.9.$$

Since the Total sum of squares is

$$S(y,y) = 6369.9,$$

the correlation ratio is $\eta^2 = 1 - 12.9/6369.9 = .998$.

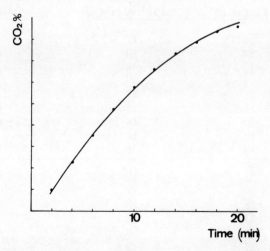

FIG. 14.8. Scatter diagram and fitted curve for data of Example 14.10.

Note: As in the case of linear regression, the regression curve is valid only for the range of values of X represented in the sample, and extrapolation outside this range may lead to erroneous conclusions. The parabola in Figure 14.8, for example, has its vertex at approximately $X = 23.3$, beyond which the values of Y decrease as X increases, and one obviously cannot assume that that portion of the curve is valid for this data.

14.6. RANK ORDER CORRELATION

It is sometimes convenient to record observations in terms of their ranks. The observations on a variable in a sample of size n would then consist of the set of ranks 1,2, . . .,n, each rank being attached to one of the sample elements. When two such variables are observed, the n observations are a set of n pairs of integers; in the ith pair, the first integer denotes the rank of the ith sample element with respect to the first variable, and thus ranges over the set 1,2, . . . , n, and the second integer denotes its rank with respect to the second variable, and is also one of the numbers 1,2, . . . , n. When two or more elements tie for the same rank, each is given a rank equal to the average of the ones that would have been assigned to them in the absence of a tie. Thus a rank may sometimes appear as a fraction. In example 14.11, for instance, one of the two cases ranked 17.5 by the first variable would have received the rank 17 and the other the rank 18 had there been no tie.

Example 14.11.   Mantel and Valand (1970) quote the rankings of a sample of size 39 (29 cancer cases and 10 controls) with respect to different measures of enzyme activity. For illustration, we take two of the enzyme determinations (labelled 2 and 3 in the original paper) as the two observed variables. The ranks for the 29 cases followed by the 10 controls are reproduced in the following table, together with the difference between the ranks for each individual.

First rank	Second rank	Difference
16	12	4
14	20	− 6
17.5	18	− .5
31.5	19	12.5
25	23	2
31.5	25	6.5
20	14	6
10	11	− 1
19	28	− 9
26	33	− 7
22	22	0
34	35	− 1
35	38	− 3
33	32	1
11	3	8
37	15.5	21.5
15	17	− 2

First rank	Second rank	Difference
39	39	0
28	31	− 3
27	29	− 2
23	30	− 7
21	26	− 5
30	27	3
13	24	− 11
24	21	3
38	36	2
29	24	5
36	37	− 1
17.5	15.5	2
8	9	− 1
5	7	− 2
9	2	7
7	10	− 3
2	4	− 2
1	6	− 5
6	8	− 2
4	1	3
3	5	− 2
12	13	− 1

One commonly used measure of association in such a sample is *Spearman's rank correlation coefficient*, which is denoted by r_s and defined as

$$r_s = 1 - \frac{6 \sum_{i=1}^{n} d_i^2}{n(n-1)(n+1)} \tag{14.18}$$

where n is the number of pairs in the sample and d_i is the difference between the ranks of the ith pair. For the data of Example 14.11, $r_s = .865$. Program REGS4 of Chapter 18 may be used to calculate r_s.

The rank correlation coefficient is very similar in nature to the correlation coefficient r of Section 14.4. In fact, if the ranks of the sample elements are considered as observations on numerical variables and Pearsons's correlation coefficient calculated from them by Formula 14.13, the result is r_s.

Like the product-moment correlation coefficient, r, the rank correlation coefficient r_s has the property that

$$-1 \leqslant r_s \leqslant + 1,$$

with the extreme values occurring in the case of perfect agreement in ranks ($r_s = + 1$) or exactly the reverse order in ranks ($r_s = -1$). The values of r_s close to zero indicate the absence of such association. To illustrate these cases, we calculate r_s in a number of different hypothetical small samples in Example 14.12.

Example 14.12   (a) Consider a sample of four elements in which the ranks given by the two variables to the elements are in perfect agreement, as in the table:

First rank	Second rank	(Difference)^2
1	1	0
4	4	0
3	3	0
2	2	0

In this case, $\Sigma\ d_i^2 = 0$, and $r_s = 1 - 0/60 = 1$.

(b) Consider now the case where the two variables rank the sample elements in exactly the opposite order from each other, as in the table:

First rank	Second rank	(Difference)^2
4	1	9
3	2	1
2	3	1
1	4	9

In this case, $\Sigma\ d_i^2 = 20$, and $r_s = 1 - 120/60 = -1$.

(c) Finally, consider the following table of ranks, in which there is neither consistent agreement nor contradiction:

First rank	Second rank	(Difference)^2
1	3	4
4	2	4
3	4	1
2	1	1

Since $\Sigma\ d_i^2 = 10$, $r_s = 1 - 6(10)/60 = 0$.

Clearly, other permutations of the ranks are possible, and the resulting values of r_s would be somewhere between -1 and $+1$.

Both the product-moment correlation coefficient r and the rank correlation coefficient r_s can be used in formal tests of the hypothesis of no association. These tests are not included in this volume, and we have limited our discussion of these two measures to their role as descriptive statistics. r_s is easier to calculate, but its main advantage lies in its versatility, as it requires no assumptions on the nature of the two variables.

14.7. MULTIPLE LINEAR REGRESSION

We have limited our discussion of regression so far to the relationship between two variables, the predictor variable X and the criterion variable Y, and we have considered the effect of X on the average value of Y as reflected in a set of bivariate data $(x_1, y_1), \ldots, (x_n, y_n)$. When Y is thought of as being affected by more than one variable factor, it is necessary to introduce additional predictor variables into the model and to consider the *joint* effect of those factors on the average value of Y. Thus, if one is to allow for the rate of growth (Y) of a guinea pig to be influenced by the animal's initial weight as well as by its food intake, the initial weight is taken as one of the predictor variables, say X_1, and a suitable measure of food intake as the other predictor variable X_2. The relationship would then be expressed in the form

$$\mu(x_1, x_2) = \alpha + \beta_1 x_1 + \beta_2 x_2 , \tag{14.19}$$

where $\mu(x_1, x_2)$ stands for the average value of Y when the variables X_1 and X_2 take the specified values x_1 and x_2, and where α, β_1 and β_2 are constants — the unknown parameters of the model.

With three variables in the model, each sample observation would consist of the three numbers (x_1, x_2, y), and the sample would therefore be a set of n triplets of this form. Instead of the scatter diagram in two dimensions, we can visualize a three-dimensional plot of the data, with X_1 and X_2 measured along the axes of a horizontal plane and Y along a vertical axis perpendicular to that plane. The result would be a set of n points suspended in space, the height of each point above or below the plane being the observed value of Y. Equation (14.19) can now be seen as the equation of a plane passing through this aggregate of points much as the regression line in two dimensions passes through the collection of points in the scatter diagram.

This geometrical interpretation of the model is necessarily more cumbersome than in the case of one predictor variable. Also, as more predictor variables are introduced into the model, the complexity of such a representation increases, and hence its usefulness as an aid in the interpretation of the methods decreases.

In general, if there are k variable factors ($k \geqslant 2$) that are possible contributors to the overall effect on a criterion variable Y, the average value of Y corresponding to a specified set of values $(x_1, \ldots, x_k)$ of the predictor variables $X_1, \ldots, X_k$ is given by the regression function

$$\mu(x_1, \ldots, x_k) = \alpha + \beta_1 x_1 + \ldots + \beta_k x_k . \tag{14.20}$$

This equation of *multiple regression* is readily seen to be an extension of Equation (14.19), in which k was equal to 2, and of Equation (14.3), in which k was only 1. A sample of n observations in this model would consist of n sets of k + 1 numbers in the order $(x_1, x_2, \ldots x_k, y)$, each set being a summary of the observations on all the variables for a single element of the sample.

As in the case of a single predictor variable (Sections 14.2 and 14.3), we shall see that a special meaning can be attached to each constant of this model, and that the constants can be estimated from the sample data by the method of least squares. The resulting equation, with the constants replaced by their estimates, can then be used in prediction. We shall also need a set of assumptions on the distributions of the variables in the model in order to make inferences about the estimates and predicted values. These extensions of the methods of earlier sections to the case of multiple regression are summarized in the following outline.

(i) *The parameters.* If the value of each X in Equation(14.20) is fixed at zero, the resulting average value of Y is α. This corresponds to the intercept in the case of k = 1, and in general it represents what can be called the "zero point" of μ, or its starting value before the effect of any of the k listed predictor variables is taken into account.

(ii) For any X_i, the coefficient β_i is the rate of change in μ with respect to X_i, while the other variables remain constant. In other words, β_i is the amount by which μ would change as a result of an increase of 1 unit in X_i and no change in any of the other X's. $\beta_1, \ldots, \beta_k$ are called *partial regression coefficients.*

(iii) *Linearity of the model.* Since μ varies at a constant rate with respect to each X_i while the other X's are held fixed, it is implied by the model that the regression of Y on each of the X_i is linear. This implication is less restrictive than it might appear, for any of the X's may be replaced in the model by its square, cube, logarithm or any function f(X) that may describe its effect on μ better than X itself. The partial regression coefficient for that X would then represent the partial change in μ *corresponding to a unit increase in f(X).* Otherwise, the model remains unaltered.

The linearity of the model is actually a characteristic of the parameters rather than the predictor variables. We note that the total effect of the X's on Y is the sum of k + 1 separate terms, each term being a multiple of one of the parameters $\alpha, \beta_1, \ldots, \beta_k$. The regression function (14.20) can therefore be seen as a linear combination of these parameters, even if each X_i is replaced by some nonlinear function $f(X_i)$.

(iv) *Polynomial models.* The variables $X_1, \ldots X_k$ need not be totally unrelated. In fact, they may be the same variable raised to different powers, as in the polynomial model

$$\mu(x) = \alpha + \beta_1 x + \beta_2 x^2 + \ldots + \beta_k x^k \;.$$

Such a model may be appropriate for *bivariate data* if the scatter diagram shows linear regression to be inappropriate while a polynomial of the second or higher degree may have a reasonably good fit (see Section 14.5.). Although each observation in such data consists only of the two numbers (x,y), the pair can be rewritten as an ordered set of k + 1 numbers $(x, x^2, \ldots x^k, y)$, and the methods of multiple linear regression can then be applied to the resulting sample. The interpretation of the partial regression coefficients must again be modified in this case.

Although a polynomial function is the most commonly used model of multiple linear regression applied to essentially bivariate data, *any* combination of functions of X may in principle replace the predictor variables, as well as combinations of powers of two or more predictors, etc.

(v) *Least squares estimates.* As in linear regression on one predictor variable, the least squares estimates of the parameters $\alpha, \beta_1, \ldots, \beta_k$ can be obtained by minimizing the sum of squared deviations

$$S = \sum_{i=1}^{n} (y_i - \mu(x_{1i}, \ldots, x_{ki}))^2$$

$$= \sum_{i=1}^{n} (y_i - \alpha - \beta_1 x_{1i} - \ldots - \beta_k x_{ki})^2 ,$$

where $(x_{1i}, \ldots, x_{ki}, y_i)$ is the ith observation in the sample. To minimize S, we must differentiate it with respect to each of the $k + 1$ parameters in turn, equate the derivatives to zero, and solve the resulting $k + 1$ simultaneous equations in the $k + 1$ unknowns $\alpha, \beta_1, \ldots, \beta_k$. Such calculations are obviously tedious, and the solutions have no simple algebraic form that is suitable for hand calculation. For a given set of data, the least squares estimates, which we denote as usual by $\hat{\alpha}, \hat{\beta}_1, \ldots \hat{\beta}_k$, can be obtained as part of the general printout of a computer program of multiple linear regression, such as those provided by SPSS and BMDP packages.

(vi) *Distribution assumptions.* For a given set of values $(x_1, \ldots, x_k)$, the criterion variable Y is assumed to be *normally distributed* with mean equal to $\mu(x_1, \ldots, x_k)$ as given in (14.20) and with variance equal to σ^2, an unknown constant which is the *same for any given set of values* $(x_1, \ldots, x_k)$.

(vii) *Estimate of the common variance.* An unbiased estimate of σ^2 is the Deviations mean square

$$s^2 = \frac{\sum_{i=1}^{n} (y_i - \hat{\alpha} - \hat{\beta}_1 x_1 - \ldots \hat{\beta}_k x_k)^2}{n - k - 1} \tag{14.21}$$

This is also given in the printout of the regression program. The denominator of the fraction in (14.21) is the number of degrees of freedom in the estimate of the variance. It is clear from this that the number of observations n must be appreciably larger than the number of predictor variables k in order for the number of degrees of freedom of the estimate to be reasonably large.

(viii) *Analysis of variance.* We denote the total sum of squared deviations of the observations on Y from their mean by S(y,y), as in previous sections. This Total sum of squares can be partitioned into two components as shown in the table:

Source of variation	Sum of squares	Degrees of freedom	Mean square
Regression		k	
Deviations	$\Sigma[y_i - \hat{\mu}(x_1, \ldots, x_k)]^2$	$n - k - 1$	s^2
Total	$S(y,y)$	$n - 1$	

where $\hat{\mu}(x_1, \ldots, x_k)$ is the regression function with the parameters replaced by their least squares estimates. This table is analogous to Table 14.1 of Section 14.3, and the mean square of deviations is again the unbiased estimate of the common variance σ^2

(ix) *Multiple correlation coefficient.* The fraction of the total variation in Y that is due to regression on the X's is denoted by R^2. That is,

$$R^2 = \frac{\text{Regression sum of squares}}{\text{Total sum of squares}} .$$

The positive square root of this ratio is *R, the coefficient of multiple correlation* between Y on the one hand and $X_1, \ldots, X_k$ on the other. This coefficient is analogous to the coefficient of linear correlation r in bivariate samples, and it can be shown to coincide with r if Y and $\beta_1 X_1 + \beta_2 X_2 + \ldots + \beta_k X_k$ are taken as the two variables.

It is easy to see that $0 \leqslant R^2 \leqslant 1$, that R is zero when the X variables have no effect at all on Y, and that it is equal to 1 in the case of perfect determination of the value of Y by the set of values of $X_1, \ldots X_k$. Unlike the correlation coefficient r, the multiple correlation coefficient R is never negative.

(x) *Partial correlation coefficients.* In addition to the multiple correlation coefficient, which is a measure of the association between Y and a combination of predictor variables, there are measures of association between *any pair* of the $k + 1$ variables while the other $k-1$ variables are held constant. These measures are known as *partial correlation coefficients.* A partial correlation coefficient is denoted by the letter r with several subscripts, the first two subscripts representing the two variables whose association is being measured, and the last string of subscripts standing for all the other variables that are held constant. Thus $r_{24.135..ky}$ is the partial correlation coefficient between X_2 and X_4, while the effect of variation in the other X's (assuming there are more than 5) and in Y is eliminated by keeping those variables constant.

REFERENCES

Abou-Daoud, K.T. (1979). *personal communication*. Department of Epidemiology and Biostatistics, American University of Beirut, Beirut, Lebanon.

Bailey, R.C., Eadie, G.S., and Schmidt, F.H. (1974). Estimation procedures for consecutive first order irreversible reactions. Biometrics, journal of The Biometric Society, *30*, 67-75.

Harakeh, M.M. (1978). Mercury content of fish and seawater in Lebanon. M.S. thesis, Department of Biology, American University of Beirut, Beirut, Lebanon.

Heller, R.F. and Jacobs, H.S. (1978). Coronary heart disease in relation to age, sex and the menopause. Br. med. J., 25 February 1978, 472-474.

Henry, J.A. and Altmann, P. (1978). Assessment of hypoproteinaemic oedema: a simple physical sign. Br. med. J., 8 April 1978, 890-891.

Hiller, R., Giacometti, L., and Yuen, K. (1977). Sunlight and cataract: an epidemiologic investigation. Am. J. Epidem. *105*, 450-459.

Mantel, N. and Valand, R.S. (1970). A technique of nonparametric multivariate analysis. Biometrics, journal of The Biometric Society, *26*, 547-558.

Sweatman, G.K. and Koussa, M.G. (1968). Comparative changes in external respiration rates of engorged *Rhipicephalus sanguineus* female ticks with age and oviposition in different physical environments. J. Parasit. *54*, 641-656.

CHAPTER 15

Validity of a Statistical Model

15.1. COMPLETELY SPECIFIED PROBABILITY MODELS

A scientific hypothesis about the source of a set of observations can sometimes be expressed in the form of a probability model, and the validity of the model can be tested by a very simple method based on the Chi-square distribution. The method is applicable equally well to observations on a qualitative or a numerical variable. Following is an outline of this procedure:

1) Given a set of n observations on a variable that can be classified into categories, and a model M specifying the probability of each category, we wish to test the hypothesis that the observations come from the distribution specified by M.

2) Let the number of categories be k, and denote the frequency observed in the ith category by O_i $(i = 1, \ldots, k)$, so that $\Sigma O_i = n$.

3) Let M specify the probability of the ith category as p_i. Then, out of the n observations, the expected frequency in the ith category is $E_i = np_i$, $i = 1, \ldots, k$. Once $E_1, \ldots, E_{k-1}$ have been calculated in this way, E_k is determined as the difference between their sum and n.

4) Calculate

$$Y = \sum_{i=1}^{k} \frac{(O_i - E_i)^2}{E_i} \tag{15.1}$$

If n is large (and not many of the E_i are very small), this statistic has approximately the Chi-square distribution with $k-1$ degrees of freedom. We note that $k-1$ was the number of expected frequencies that had to be calculated from the model.

5) Find the significant values of the χ^2_{k-1} variable corresponding to an arbitrary significance level α, and reject the hypothesis tested if

$$Y > \chi^2_{k-1}(\alpha). \tag{15.2}$$

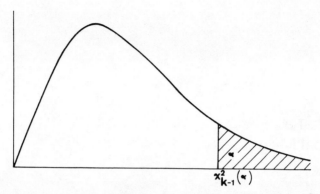

FIG. 15.1. Upper percentile of the Chi-square distribution with k−1 d.f.

Example 15.1. In an investigation of the theory of biorhythm and its possible relation to highway crashes, Shaffer *et al* (1978) identified the "plus" and "minus" periods in the biorhythm cycles of the motorists who were clearly at fault in 153 fatal or at least serious accidents. With three biocycles (P, S and I) defined for each person, there are 8 combinations of "plus" and "minus" periods. The authors' hypothesis is that there is no relation between the cycles and accident likelihood, so that the driver is as likely to belong to any one of the 8 combinations as any other. Therefore $p_i = .125$ for $i = 1, \ldots, 8$, and since $n = 153$ the expected frequencies E_i are each equal to $(153)(.125) = 19.125$, as shown in Table 15.1. The corresponding observed frequencies are also shown in the table.

Table 15.1. Comparison of observed and expected frequencies in Example 15.1

Biorhythm Cycles			Observed Frequency	Expected Frequency
P	S	I		
+	+	+	15	19.125
+	+	−	25	19.125
+	−	+	23	19.125
+	−	−	18	19.125
−	+	+	21	19.125
−	+	−	16	19.125
−	−	+	16	19.125
−	−	−	19	19.125
Total			153	153.000

Source : Shaffer *et al* (1978). Copyright 1978 American Medical Association

The value of Y calculated from this table is 4.75. This has a P–value of about 0.69, therefore the hypothesis would be accepted at any of the conventional levels.

Example 15.2. This example considers a hypothetical set of survival data in which the variable is numerical and the categories are not initially defined. Let the variable be survival in years after treatment, and suppose that, according to the model M, this variable has the exponential distribution with mean $\mu = 1/2$ (see Section 4.4 d). With this model, the probabilities of different intervals of x values can be obtained in two ways: one is by integration of the density function, which leads to the cumulative probability $P(X \leqslant x) = 1 - e^{-x/2}$; the other is by recognizing this particular exponential distribution as identical with χ_2^2 (see Section 4.4 e), and using the table of Chi-square probabilities. In either case, we find that more than 90% of the values of X in this model are under 5, so we consider the six intervals shown in Table 15.2 as the categories of classification. If the range of likely values of X under the hypothesis tested were larger than 5, we would have defined the categories as wider time intervals. The number of categories for such a variable is obviously quite arbitrary, but care must be taken that the division does not result in several very small expected frequencies. To test the validity of this model for a set of 100 hypothetical observations, we classify our observations in the 6 categories and obtain the column of observed frequencies, O_i, in Table 15.2. The column of expected frequencies, E_i, is obtained by multiplying each category probability by 100. Taking a significance level of 10 percent, we calculate Y by Formula (15.1) and apply the criterion (15.2) in which $\chi_5^2 (.10) = 9.24$. Since $Y = 16.19$, we reject the hypothesis that this model is appropriate for our data.

Table 15.2. Comparison of observed and expected
frequencies in Example 15.2

Interval i	P(X in interval i)	E_i	O_i
0 – 1⁻	.3935	39.35	25
1 – 2⁻	.2386	23.86	35
2 – 3⁻	.1448	14.48	15
3 – 4⁻	.0878	8.78	10
4 – 5⁻	.0532	5.32	10
5 – 9⁻	.0821	8.21	5

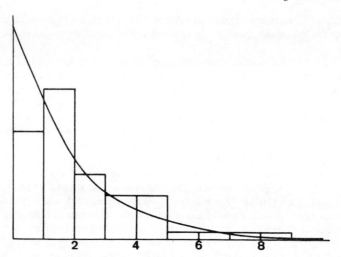

FIG. 15.2.   Observed (histogram) and expected (areas under curve) frequencies in Example 15.2.

15.2. FITTING A THEORICAL DISTRIBUTION

The models considered in the previous section assigned a numerical value to the probability of each category, so that all the p_i were completely specified. This is not always the case. More often than not, a model would give the observed variable a certain *type* of distribution, leaving one or more of the parameters unspecified, so that the p_i, which depend on the unknown parameters, are also unknown. To test the validity of such a model, we first seek from among all the distributions of the type given by the model the one that best describes the observations; this is done by using the given observations to estimate the unknown parameters of the distribution. Once a particular distribution of that type is identified, the p_i of the different categories are calculated, and the method of the previous section is applied. Following is an outline of the procedure:

1) Given a set of n observations on a numerical variable X (continuous or discrete) and a model M stating that X has a distribution of a certain type (normal, or Poisson, or exponential, etc.) but with unknown parameters, we wish to test the hypothesis that the observations come from such a distribution.

2) Suppose that the distribution type given by M has m unknown parameters ($m \geqslant 1$). Using the given n observations, find estimates of these parameters in the usual way and replace each unknown parameter by its estimate. The resulting distribution is called the "best-fitting" distribution of the given type.

3) Define k categories for the values of X and denote the frequency observed in the ith category by O_i (i = 1, . . . k), so that $\Sigma\, O_i = n$.

4) Let the probability assigned to the ith category by the best-fitting distribution be p_i. Then, out of the n observations, the expected frequency in the ith category is $E_i = np_i$ $(i = 1, \ldots k)$. As in the previous section, only $k-1$ of these expected frequencies need to be calculated from the model, the kth being the difference between their sum and n.

5) Calculate

$$Y = \sum_{i=1}^{k} \frac{(O_i - E_i)^2}{E_i} .$$ (15.3)

If n is large (and not many of the E_i are very small), this statistic has approximately the Chi-square distribution with $k-1-m$ degrees of freedom. We note that the degrees of freedom of this statistic are fewer than those of the statistic defined in Formula (15.1) by m, which is the number of estimated parameters. In effect, each parameter estimated has imposed an additional restriction on the data and thus decreases the number of degrees of freedom by 1.

6) At significance level α, reject the hypothesis that the observations come from the given type of distribution if

$$Y > \chi^2_{k-1-m}(\alpha).$$ (15.4)

This rule is based on the argument that, if the best-fitting distribution of the type given by M does not describe the data sufficiently well, no other distribution of that type would do so.

The method outlined above is known as testing the *goodness of fit* of a distribution.

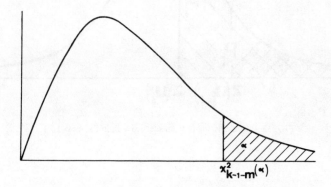

FIG. 15.3. Upper percentile of the Chi-square distribution with k-1-m d.f.

Example 15.3. To illustrate the above procedure, we test the goodness of fit of a normal distribution to the data of Example 7.1 (p. 87), which contains 51 observations on the calcium content (in mg/1) in water samples. We follow the same sequence as in the steps outlined above.

1) In this example, n = 51, and the distribution type is normal.

2) We estimate the mean and standard deviation of the best-fitting normal distribution as $\hat{\mu} = \overline{X} = 62.92$ and $\hat{\sigma} = s = 17.90$. In this example, m = 2.

3) A quick look at the data suggests that a convenient division of the values of X into categories is by class intervals of 10 units' width, as in column (1) of Table 15.3, where l_i refers to the lower, and u_i to the upper, limit of the ith class interval. The observed frequencies are given in column (6).

4) Using the estimates of the parameters, we standardize the upper limit of each class interval, except the last (which contains all values of X in the right tail, while the first interval contains all values in the left tail). For the ith interval, the standardized upper limit is $z(u_i) = (u_i - \overline{X})/s$ and is shown in column (2) in the table. Using a table of normal probabilities (Table II in the Appendix) we calculate $P_i = P(Z \leqslant z(u_i))$ for each class interval except the last and record these cumulative probabilities in column (3). Then p_i is the difference between the ith and (i−1)st entries of this column, as can be seen from Figure 15.4. The expected frequencies are now calculated as $E_i = (51)p_i$ and entered in column (5).

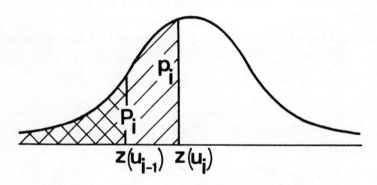

FIG. 15.4. Calculating p_i from successive P_i in Example 15.3.

5) Using columns (5) and (6), we calculate Y by Formula (15.3) and find that Y = 4.51.

6) We have k = 8 and m = 2. Therefore, if $\alpha = .05$, we compare the calculated Y with $\chi_5^2 (.05) = 11.071$. Since Y is smaller, we accept the hypothesis that the normal model provides a good fit for the data at this level.

Table 15.3. Fitting a normal distribution to data of
Examples 7.1 and 15.3

(1) $l_i - u_i^-$	(2) $z(u_i)$	(3) P_i	(4) p_i	(5) E_i	(6) O_i
$-\infty - 30^-$	-1.84	0.0329	0.0329	1.68	1
$30 - 40^-$	-1.28	0.1003	0.0674	3.44	3
$40 - 50^-$	-0.72	0.2358	0.1355	6.91	8
$50 - 60^-$	-0.16	0.4364	0.2006	10.23	10
$60 - 70^-$	0.39	0.6554	0.2190	11.17	13
$70 - 80^-$	0.95	0.8289	0.1735	8.85	5
$80 - 90^-$	1.51	0.9345	0.1056	5.39	6
$90 - \infty$		1.0000	0.0655	3.34	5

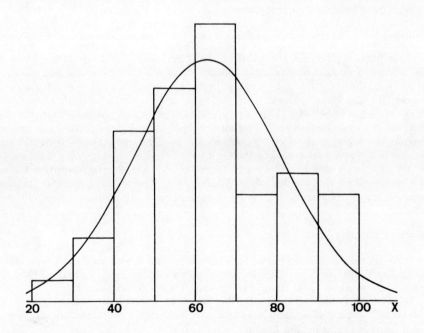

FIG. 15.5. Observed (histogram) and expected (areas under curve) frequencies in Example 15.3.

It is easy to see how the same method that was used with the normal distribution in the above example can also be used with any theoretical distribution whose parameters are readily estimated. One class of distributions which is sometimes of interest in biological experiments, and for which the estimation of parameters may cause difficulties in carrying out the goodness of fit test, is the class of *truncated* distributions. A distribution is truncated if some values of the variable in the right or left tail, or both, are simply not observed. For example, Holgate (1966) considered three possible discrete distributions as models for his data on the number of captures in a trapping experiment. Since only those animals that were captured one or more times could be observed, the distributions were truncated below 1, or "zero-truncated".

Estimation in truncated normal distributions is discussed by Bliss (1967, ch. 7). References to various results on the estimation of parameters in truncated distributions can be found in Kendall and Stuart (1967, ch. 32).

15.3.   QUICK TESTS OF NORMALITY

Since the normal distribution is at the basis of most of our statistical methods of analysis, its validity as a model for a given set of data is a matter that is very frequently investigated. We have already seen that this investigation can be carried out formally by means of the technique of the previous section. However, departures from normality can also be detected by less elaborate methods, of which we mention the following:

Skewness

If the frequency polygon constructed from a large sample is clearly skewed, this is an indication of lack of normality in the population, and a formal test of the goodness of fit of a normal distribution is not necessary. In this connection, it must be pointed out that a symmetrical frequency polygon is not necessarily an indication of normality, since some of the symmetrical bell-shaped density curves are more peaked and some more flat than the normal curve. Skewness can, of course, be present in various degrees, and one can measure the degree of skewness by calculating a "coefficient of skewness" from the sample, but that is no longer a quick method.

If a distribution appears to be highly skewed to the right, the transformation $Y = \log X$ if all the values of X are positive, or $Y = \log (X + c)$ if all the values of X are larger than $-c$, where c is positive, has the effect of bringing the distribution closer to the normal.

Normal Probability Paper

These are special graph sheets with an arithmetical horizontal scale and a vertical probability scale. The vertical scale is marked in such a way that a set of pairs $(x, P(X \leqslant x))$ plotted on this paper would fall on a straight line if X is a normal variable.

To check on the normality of a variable in a set of observations, we classify the observations in a frequency distribution and plot, for each class interval, the cumulative relative frequency (up to and including that class) against the upper boundary of the interval. If the points fall more or less along a straight line, we can accept the data as originating from a normal population.

Probits

This is essentially the same method as the one mentioned in the previous paragraph, except that it requires no special graph paper. A table of *probits* is convenient but not necessary, as the values can be read directly from a table of probabilities of the standard normal variable Z. Corresponding to a relative frequency R, the probit is defined as (5) + (the percentile of Z below which the probability is R). That is, $P(Z \leqslant \text{Probit}(R) - 5) = R$, as in Figure 15.6. A table of probits, such as Table XI 1 in Fisher and Yates (1974) facilitates the calculations.

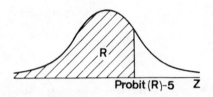

FIG. 15.6. The probit corresponding to proportion R.

If the probits of several values of a normal variable are plotted with the values as abscissae and the probits as ordinates, the points fall on a straight line. Therefore, to test for normality from a set of data classified in a frequency distribution we transform the relative cumulative frequency of each class interval into its probit and plot the points (upper limit of interval, probit) on ordinary graph paper. If the points fall more or less along a straight line, the data is assumed to come from a normal population.

Example 15.4. In this example, we apply the probit method to the frequency distribution of Example 15.3. We first calculate the cumulative frequency F_i and the cumulative relative frequency R_i for each of the class intervals, as in the third and fourth columns of Table 15.4. To calculate the probit corresponding to each R_i, we first find the value of Z below which the area under the standard normal curve is R_i (using Table II of the Appendix). Add 5 to this value of Z, and the result is the probit.

In Figure 15.7, we have plotted the 7 points each having as abscissa the upper class boundary and as ordinate the probit corresponding to that boundary. The points appear to fall along a straight line, which supports the hypothesis of normality for the population from which this data originated.

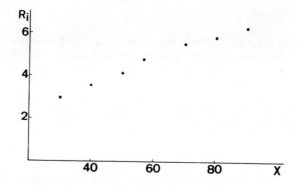

FIG. 15.7.   Probits for data of Examples 7.1 and 15.3.

Table 15.4.   Probits for data of Examples 7.1 and 15.3

Class interval			O_i	F_i	R_i	Probit(R_i)
$-\infty$	$-$	30^-	1	1	0.0196	2.94
30	$-$	40^-	3	4	0.0784	3.58
40	$-$	50^-	8	12	0.2353	4.28
50	$-$	60^-	10	22	0.4314	4.83
60	$-$	70^-	13	35	0.6863	5.49
70	$-$	80^-	5	40	0.7843	5.79
80	$-$	90^-	6	46	0.9020	6.29
90	$-$	∞	5	51	1.0000	

REFERENCES

Bliss, C.I. (1967). *Statistics in Biology,* vol. I, McGraw Hill, New York.

Fisher, R.A. and Yates, F. (1974). *Statistical Tables for Biological, Agricultural and Medical Research*, 6th ed., (Longman, London).

Holgate, P. (1966). Contributions to the mathematics of animal trapping. Biometrics, journal of The Biometric Society, *22*, 925-936.

Kendall, M.G. and Stuart, A. (1967). *The Advanced Theory of Statistics*, vol II, 2nd ed., Charles Griffin and Co., London.

Shaffer, J.W., Schmidt, C.W., Zlotowitz, H.I, and Fisher, R.S. (1978). Biorhythms and highway crashes. Are they related? Archives of General Psychiatry *35*, 41-46.

CHAPTER 16

Comparing Two Unspecified Distributions

16.1. INTRODUCTION

On several occasions in previous chapters, our problem was to test the equality of a certain parameter for a specified type of distribution in two different populations. Thus, the proportions in two binomial populations were compared in Chapter 12, the standard deviations of two normal populations were compared in Chapter 11, and the means (with equal or unequal standard deviations) in Chapter 9. In this chapter, the distributions in the two populations will be compared without reference to any particular parameter, and the methods used in this comparison are called *nonparametric methods*. With nonparametric methods, the type of distribution need not be specified either, and the methods are applicable equally well to any discrete or continuous variable with any distribution. For this reason, they are also known as *distribution-free* methods. Besides avoiding the need to make assumptions on the distribution of the variable, these methods have the advantage of being, in general, easier to apply, requiring as they do fewer calculations than the standard tests based on the normal assumptions.

Given two samples, the problem is to test the hypothesis that, in the two populations from which the samples were taken, the observed variable has exactly the same (unspecified) distribution. As for alternative hypotheses, the types usually considered are alternatives of shift in location; that is, the alternative may claim that the first population values are in general larger than the second (right-sided alternatives), that they are in general smaller than the second (left-sided alternatives), or that they are in general not equal to those of the second (two-sided alternatives). Several tests have been developed for these problems, and we shall describe and illustrate four of them in the following sections. Two will be presented separately for use with paired samples, and the other two for use with independent samples. For a discussion on the distinction between the two types of samples, see Section 9.1.

16.2. PAIRED SAMPLES

Given two paired (or matched) samples, each consisting of n observations on a numerical variable X, let $D_1, \ldots, D_n$ represent the n sample differences: D_i = (ith observation from population I) minus (corresponding observation from population II), for $i = 1, \ldots, n$. The problem is to test the hypothesis

H_0 : The variable X has the same distribution in the two populations,

at some given significance level α.

As alternative hypotheses, we consider any of the following:

H_R : The values of X in population I are in general larger (right-sided alternatives),

H_L : The values of X in population I are in general smaller (left-sided alternatives),

H_T : The values of X in population I are either larger or smaller (two-sided alternatives).

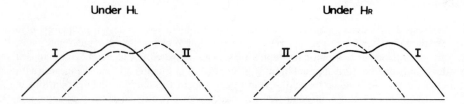

FIG. 16.1.   The two populations under H_L and H_R.

16.2 a. The Sign Test

The Sign Test has already been used in a different context in Chapter 8. Its application in this problem is similar.

1) We first calculate the differences $D_1, \ldots, D_n$. If any of these differences is zero, we eliminate the pair of equal observations from the sample, since no information is provided by it about differences between the populations. Then the *sample size* n *is taken as the number of non-zero differences.*

2) If H_0 is true, $P(\text{any } D_i > 0) = P(\text{any } D_i < 0) = 0.5$. Define

$$R = \text{number of positive } D_i. \tag{16.1}$$

Then R, which is a binomial variable with parameters n and 0.5, is the test statistic.

3) Since R is the number of positive differences, large values of R support H_R, small values of R support H_L, and in testing against the two-sided alternative H_T the significant values of R are in the two tails of the distribution.

4) If $n \geqslant 10$, R is approximately normal with mean $\mu = n/2$ and standard deviation $\sigma = \sqrt{n}/2$. With the correction for continuity, the significant values of the standardized R are as follows:

(i) $\dfrac{2R - n - 1}{\sqrt{n}} > z(\alpha)$

when testing against H_R;

(ii) $\dfrac{2R - n + 1}{\sqrt{n}} < -z(\alpha)$ (16.2)

when testing against H_L;

(iii) $\dfrac{|2R - n| - 1}{\sqrt{n}} > z(\alpha/2)$

when testing against H_T.

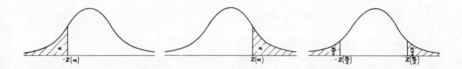

FIG. 16.2. Percentiles of the standard normal distribution

Example 16.1. In a study of diurnal variation in plasma cortisol levels, Yerevanian *et al* (1975) determined 8 a.m. and 8 p.m. levels for different groups of subjects. Their figures for 11 patients with Cushing's syndrome are reproduced in columns 2 and 3 of Table 16.1.

Since $D = 0$ for one of the patients, the number of pairs n is reduced to 10. The signs of the 10 differences, "8 a.m. level" minus "8 p.m. level", are entered in the fourth column of Table 16.1. The last two columns will not be used in this example.

We now apply the Sign Test to the hypothesis that the distribution of plasma cortisol levels is the same at 8 a.m. and 8 p.m. in this group of subjects, against the alternative that the 8 a.m. level is higher (as is the case with normal subjects). From the table, we see that $R = 4$, and this is clearly not significant in testing against the right-sided alternative at the usual levels. In fact, the P–value of the calculated R is $P(Z \geqslant -3/\sqrt{10}) = .83$.

Table 16.1. Nonparametric tests for paired samples

Plasma Cortisol $\mu g/100$ ml

Patient	8 a.m.	8 p.m.	Sign of D	|D|	Signed Rank |D|
1	16.5	13.8	+	2.7	8
2	10.0	9.9	+	0.1	1
3	16.4	16.7	−	0.3	− 3.5
4	22.0	22.5	−	0.5	− 5
5	34.5	34.5	+	10.0	10
6	9.0	9.3	−	0.3	− 3.5
7	12.6	12.8	−	0.2	− 2
8	12.7	11.5	+	1.2	7
9	12.0	15.5	−	3.5	−9
10	9.9	11.0	−	1.1	−6
11	59.0	59.0	0		

$$R = 4 \qquad\qquad T = 26$$

Source : Yerevanian *et al* (1975)

This test can be carried out by means of Program SIGNT of Chapter 18.

16.2 b. The Signed Ranks Test

This test, which is due to Wilcoxon (1945), makes more use of the data than the Sign Test does, as it takes into account the magnitudes of the differences as well as their signs.

Again consider using a set of n positive or negative differences between paired observations to test the hypothesis H_0 against any of the three possible types of alternatives at significance level α.

1) Ignoring the signs of the differences D_i, assign ranks to their magnitudes $|D_i|$, starting with 1 for the smallest of these quantities. In the case of "ties", that is if two or more of the $|D_i|$ are equal, each of the tied quantities is assigned the same rank, which is the average of the ranks that would have been assigned in the absence of a tie. For example, if two $|D_i|$ tie for the fourth place, each is given the rank 4.5.

2) The rank of each of the $|D_i|$ is now given the sign of the original difference , so that the result is a set of n "signed ranks".

3) Calculate the sum of the positive ranks and that of the negative ranks. Clearly, if H_0 is true, the two sums should be approximately equal and, since the sum of *all* the n ranks is n (n + 1) /2, each of the separate sums should be close to half this amount, or n (n +|1)//4. If H_0 is not true, one of the sums is appreciably smaller and the other appreciably| larger. Thus a reasonable test statistic is:

$$T = \text{sum of positive ranks.} \tag{16.3}$$

The exact distribution of this statistic was derived by Wilcoxon (1945), and tables of its probabilities are available in various sources (see, for instance. Table 23 in Pearson and Hartley, 1972, Table A9 in Snedecor and Cochran, 1967, or Table C11 in Brown and Hollander, 1977). These tables need not be used unless n is very small. For large n (say $\geqslant$ 10), an approximate test based on the standardized statistic T is fairly accurate.

4) When the number of pairs is large, T is approximately normally distributed under H_0, with $\mu = n(n + 1)/4$ and $\sigma = \sqrt{n(n+1)(2n+1)/24}$, so that the standardized statistic T, with the correction for continuity, becomes $(T - \mu \pm 0.5)/\sigma$, and the test consists of rejecting H_0 at level α if

$$\text{(i)} \frac{2T - n(n+1)/2 - 1}{\sqrt{n(n+1)(2n+1)/6}} > z(\alpha)$$

when testing against H_R ; or if

$$\text{(ii)} \frac{2T - n(n+1)/2 + 1}{\sqrt{n(n+1)(2n+1)/6}} < -z(\alpha) \tag{16.4}$$

when testing against H_L ; or if

$$\text{(iii)} \frac{|2T - n(n+1)/2| - 1}{\sqrt{n(n+1)(2n+1)/6}} > z(\alpha/2)$$

when testing against H_T .

Example 16.2. We return to the data of Example 16.1 and prepare the way for calculating the statistic T by completing the last two columns of Table 16.1. These entries were obtained according to Steps 1 and 2 in the above procedure. Adding the positive signed ranks, we get $T = 26$.

To apply the approximate test, we take a right-sided alternative, as in Example 16.1. Here, the rule is to reject H_0 in favor of H_R if the standardized T is too large. Let $\alpha = .05$, then $z(.05) = 1.645$. Since the standardized T is $(52 - 55 - 1)/\sqrt{385} = -.2039$, which is far below 1.645, we accept H_0.

It is easy to see in this example, as in Example 16.1, that H_0 would have been accepted in testing against a left-handed alternative as well.

It may be instructive to compare the significant values of T in the approximate and exact tests for $n = 10$ and $\alpha = .05$. By the approximate test, values of

$$\frac{T - 28}{\sqrt{96.25}} > 1.645$$

are significant. This implies that the significant values of the unstandardized T are

$$T > 1.645\sqrt{96.25} + 28 = 44.14$$

or that the P–value of 44.14 is .05. From Table C11 in Brown and Hollander (1977), we find that the P–value of $44 = .053$, and the P–value of $45 = .042$. Therefore, at the 5% level, the significant values of the test statistic T, which is a discrete variable, are those in which T is 45 or more, the same in both tests.

16.3. INDEPENDENT SAMPLES

We now suppose that a sample of size n_1 is taken from the first population and, quite independently, a sample of size n_2 is taken from the second. The object is again to test the hypothesis that the variable observed has the same distribution in the two populations. As in the previous section, we denote this hypothesis by H_0 and the three types of alternative hypotheses by H_R, H_L and H_T.

Two tests of H_0 will be given below. Both are based on the argument that, if the n_1 and n_2 observations are mixed together and arranged in ascending order, the observations from one of the samples should alternate with those from the other in random fashion if H_0 is true, or tend to cluster at one end of the sequence if H_R or H_L is true. To distinguish the elements of the two samples in the mixture, we denote the observations from the first population by $X_1, \ldots, X_{n_1}$ and those from the second by $Y_1, \ldots, Y_{n_2}$. It must be remembered, however, that X and Y stand for the same kind of variable; in fact, if H_0 is true, they *are* the same variable.

16.3 a. The Median Test

Suppose that the observations from the two samples have been arranged in ascending order and marked in such a way that each element is identified as belonging to one or the other of the samples.

1) Let C be the median of the combined sample. If $n_1 + n_2$ is even, C is any number between the two observations at the centre of the sequence; if $n_1 + n_2$ is odd, C is the central observation. In either case, the number of observations that are smaller than C is $[(n_1 + n_2)/2]$ where the symbol [a number] stands for "the largest integer contained in that number". Call this quantity h. Then h is half the combined sample size if the combined sample size is even, or the integer just below the half if the combined sample size is odd.

2) Define a test statistic R as follows:

$$R = \text{the number of X's smaller than the common median C.} \tag{16.5}$$

If H_0 is true, R should have a value near $n_1/2$. In general, R is an integer between 0 and h, with a large R implying generally smaller values of the X's, and vice versa.

3) In view of the above, in testing H_0 against H_R (X's in general larger than Y's), small values of R are significant; in testing against H_L (X's in general smaller than Y's), large values of R are significant; and in testing against H_T, extreme values of R (near 0 or h) are significant.

4) The probability distribution of R, under H_0, is known to be

$$P(R = r) = \frac{n_1!\, n_2!\, h!\, (n_1 + n_2 - h)!}{r!\, (n_1 - r)!\, (h-r)!\, (n_2 - h + r)!\, (n_1 + n_2)!} \tag{16.6}$$

for $r = 0, 1, 2, ..., n$ or h (whichever is smaller), and where k! stands for the *factorial of k*, which is defined as $k(k-1)(k-2) \ldots (3)(2)(1)$ for any positive integer k, and $0! = 1$. This formula can be used to calculate the P−value of any observed r.

5) When $n_1 + n_2$ is large, R is approximately normal with mean $\mu = hn_1/(n_1 + n_2)$ and variance $\sigma^2 = n_1 n_2 h\, (n_1 + n_2 - h)/[(n_1 + n_2)^2(n_1 + n_2 - 1)]$. Therefore the standardized R is

$$Z = \frac{(n_1 + n_2)R - hn_1}{\sqrt{n_1 n_2 h\, (n_1 + n_2 - h)/(n_1 + n_2 - 1)}}. \tag{16.7}$$

6) If the two original *samples are of equal sizes,* that is if $n_1 = n_2$, Formulas (16.6) and (16.7) become much simpler in form. Denoting the sample size of each sample by n, we see that h is also equal to n and (16.6) reduces to

$$P(R = r) = \frac{(n!)^4}{[r!\, (n-r)!]^2\, (2n)!} \tag{16.8}$$

while (16.7) reduces to

$$Z = \frac{(2R-n)\sqrt{2n-1}}{n}. \tag{16.9}$$

7) Now the large-sample test is as follows: R is significant at level α if

(i) $Z < -z(\alpha)$ when testing against H_R; or

(ii) $Z > z(\alpha)$ when testing against H_L; or $\tag{16.10}$

(iii) $|Z| > z(\alpha/2)$ when testing against H_T.

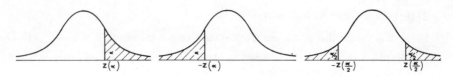

FIG. 16.3. Percentiles of the standard normal distribution

Example 16.3. In Example 9.5 (p. 114), the data consisted of two independent samples of size 10 each. The observations were

$$X - 12.0 \quad 0.0 \quad 9.3 \quad 8.1 \quad 5.8 \quad 6.8 \quad 3.6 \quad 9.5 \quad 8.6 \quad 7.3$$
$$Y - 5.8 \quad 0.0 \quad 7.0 \quad 0.0 \quad 7.5 \quad 2.6 \quad 5.5 \quad 7.2 \quad 7.3 \quad 3.3$$

We use this data to test the hypothesis H_0 against the two-sided alternative H_T. Since $n_1 = n_2$, we use Formula (16.8) for the exact test and Formula (16.9) for the approximate test. The combined sample, rearranged in ascending order and with the X observations underlined, is as follows:

<u>0.0</u>   0.0   0.0   2.6   3.3   <u>3.6</u>   5.5   <u>5.8</u>   5.8   <u>6.8</u>

7.0   7.2   7.3   <u>7.3</u>   7.5   <u>8.1</u>   <u>8.6</u>   <u>9.3</u>   <u>9.5</u>   <u>12.0</u>

The median C of the combined sample is between 6.8 and 7.0, and R = 4.

(a) To calculate the P–value of the observed R, we recall that the alternative is two-sided, and therefore the P–value is the probability, under H_0, of R being as far from its expected value *in either direction* as 4, or farther. Since the expected value is $\mu = 5$,

$$\begin{aligned}
\text{P–value of } 4 &= P(R \leqslant 4 \quad \text{or} \quad R \geqslant 6) \\
&= 1 - P(R = 5) \\
&= 1 - .34, \quad \text{using Formula (16.8)} \\
&= .66.
\end{aligned}$$

(b) Take $\alpha = .05$. The standardized value of 4 is, by Formula (16.9), $Z = -2\sqrt{19}/10 = -.87$. But $z(.025) = 1.96$. Since $|-.87| < 1.96$, we accept H_0 against H_T at the 5% level.

The *approximate* P–value of the observed R is $P(|Z| \geqslant .87) = 2(.3078) = .6156$.

Example 16.4. To illustrate the calculations when the sample sizes are not equal, we use the data of Example 9.6 to test H_0 against the right-sided alternative H_R at the .01 level. The samples were:

X $-$	16.1	16.8	13.5	13.0	14.3	11.6	12.8	17.5	12.8
	8.9	16.0	16.8	16.7	15.2				
Y $-$	14.6	11.1	7.0	10.4	15.8	14.6	9.4	9.8	5.1
	5.5	6.4	7.1						

so that $n_1 = 14$, $n_2 = 12$, and therefore $h = 13$. The combined sample, with X values underlined, is as follows:

5.1	5.5	6.4	7.0	7.1	8.9	9.4
9.8	10.4	11.1	11.6	12.8	12.8	13.0
13.5	14.3	14.6	14.6	15.2	15.8	16.0
16.1	16.7	16.8	16.8	17.5		

We immediately see that C is between 12.8 and 13.0 and that $R = 4$.

(a) Although the combined sample is large enough for the normal approximation, we show here how to calculate the P$-$value of the observed R by the exact method.

Since the alternative is right-sided, the significant values of R are the small ones, and therefore the P$-$value is $P(R \leqslant 4)$ under H_0. Substituting for n_1, n_2 and h in Formula (16.6), we get

$$P(R = r) = \frac{14! \; 12! \; (13!)^2}{26! \; r!(14-r)!(13-r)!(-1+r)!} \; .$$

We notice that, with $n_1 > h$, it is impossible for R to be zero. Therefore $P(R \leqslant 4)$ $= P(R = 1) + P(R = 2) + P(R = 3) + P(R = 4) = .0000 + .0001 + .0023 + .0212$ $= .0236$.

(b) For the approximate test, we standardize, R, using $\mu = (13)(14)/26 = 7$ and $\sigma = \sqrt{(12)(14)(13)(26-13)/[(26)(26)(25)]} = 1.30$. Therefore $Z = -2.31$. Since the significant values of Z are those smaller than $-z(.01) = -2.326$, we accept H_0. At a higher significance level, like 5% or even 2%, we would have rejected the hypothesis tested, since the calculated Z is very small. In fact, the approximate P$-$value of R is $P(R \leqslant 4) = P(Z \leqslant -2.31) = .0104$.

16.3 b. The Rank Sum Test

This test, also known as the Mann-Whitney-Wilcoxon test, can be based on any one of several test statistics, all of which are related and lead to the same conclusion. We shall use what is called the U-statistic.

1) Again suppose that the observations from the two samples have been combined and arranged in ascending order. For each Y in the combined sample, count the number of X observations that are smaller than it.Then add up these counts for all the Y's, and call the sum U. That is,

$$U = \text{the number of pairs (X,Y) in which } X < Y. \tag{16.11}$$

To keep track of the counts, it is advisable to start with, say, the largest Y, count the X's below it, then take the next largest and count the X's below it, etc.

2) If all the X's are larger than all the Y's, $U = 0$. At the other extreme, if all the X's are smaller than all the Y's, then each of the n_2 Y's has n_1 X's below it, and the total count is $n_1 n_2$. Therefore $0 \leqslant U \leqslant n_1 n_2$, with small values of U supporting the alternative H_R and large values supporting H_L; intermediate values of U are likely to occur when the two samples are well mixed in the combined sample, and such values would therefore support H_0.

3) If n_1 and n_2 are large, the statistic U has, under H_0, a distribution which is approximately normal with mean equal to $\mu = n_1 n_2/2$ and standard deviation equal to $\sigma = \sqrt{n_1 n_2 (n_1 + n_2 + 1)/12}$. Therefore the standardized U is

$$Z = \frac{U - n_1 n_2/2}{\sqrt{n_1 n_2 (n_1 + n_2 + 1)/12}}. \tag{16.12}$$

4) For testing H_0 at level α, we consider U significant if

(i) $Z < -z(\alpha)$ when testing against H_R; or

(ii) $Z > z(\alpha)$ when testing against H_L; or $\tag{16.13}$

(iii) $|Z| > z(\alpha/2)$ when testing against the two-sided alternative H_T.

Example 16.5. We return to the data of Example 9.6 which was used in Example 16.4 above. In this example, $n_1 = 14$ and $n_2 = 12$. Therefore, if H_0 is true, the statistic U has mean $\mu = 84$ and standard deviation $\sigma = 19.44$. We refer to the combined sample listed in Example 16.4 and, starting with the largest Y, we find that $Y = 15.8$ has 8 X's below it, $Y = 14.6$ has 7 X's below it, the other $Y = 14.6$ has 7 X's below it, etc., making a total of 26 times that an X appears below a Y. Therefore $U = 26$. Standardizing U, we have $Z = (26 - 84)/19.44 = -2.98$.Since the significant values of Z are those smaller than $-z(.01) = -2.326$, we reject H_0 at this level.

REFERENCES

Brown, B.W. and Hollander, M. (1977). *Statistics: A Biomedical Introduction.* Wiley, New York.

Pearson, E.S. and Hartley, H.O. (editors). (1972). *Biometrika Tables for Statisticians,* vol. II. Cambridge University Press, Cambridge, England.

Snedecor, G.W. and Cochran, W.G. (1967). *Statistical Methods,* 6th ed., Iowa State University Press. Ames, Iowa, U.S.A.

Wilcoxon, F. (1945). Individual comparisons by ranking methods. Biometrics Bulletin *1,* 80-83.

Yerevanian, B.I., Wehby, V.S., and Salti, I.S. (1975). The diagnostic value of plasma cortisol in adrenocortical disorders. J. med. liban. *28,* 415-438.

CHAPTER 17
Some Misuses of Statistics

In this chapter, we cite some of the more common examples of statistical malpractice that have been encountered by the authors in their reading and consulting experience. The list includes typical pitfalls in the application of standard statistical techniques and in the interpretation of results, but is by no means exhaustive. To minimize calculations and bring out the essential point of each example, we have kept sample sizes small and used hypothetical data of unrealistic numerical simplicity.

Example 17.1. (Chi-Square)

Question: Suppose that a patient in a certain condition is expected to spend 15 days in recovery. A sample of 6 patients were observed to recover after

19   18   22   6   19   12

days. Is this consistent with our expectation? Take $\alpha = .05$.

Incorrect analysis: For the 6 subjects, we have the observed and expected number of days as follows:

Subject	Observed	Expected
1	19	15
2	18	15
3	22	15
4	6	15
5	19	15
6	12	15

Therefore, by Formula (15.1), $Y = \Sigma \ (O - E)^2 /E = 12$. Since $\chi^2_5 (.05) = 11.07$, we find Y significant at the 5% level and conclude that the observations do not fit the model.

Comment: The observed *variable* (number of days) *is not qualitative* and the figures appearing under O and E in the above table are not frequencies. Therefore the Chi-square test of fit is not appropriate.

The problem in fact concerns testing the value of a population mean, namely testing $H_0 : \mu = 15$ against $H_T : \mu \neq 15$ on the basis of a sample of size 6. We calculate $\overline{X} = 16$ and $s = 5.9$ from the 6 observations and find, by Formula (8.16), that the standardized sample mean is $T_0 = 0.415$, which is certainly not significant at the 5% level. Its P–value, read from tables of the t–distribution more extensive than our Table IV, is over 72%. The hypothesis is therefore accepted.

Example 17.2. (Two means)

Question: Seven subjects were observed before and after a certain treatment which is supposed to increase the subject's response to a stimulus, with the object of determining whether the treatment has any effect on the average response. That is, the problem is to test the hypothesis $H_0 : \mu_B - \mu_A = 0$ against $H_L : \mu_B - \mu_A < 0$ on the basis of the observations

Before	After
10	12
15	18
22	21
8	10
12	15
20	22
5	8

Take $\alpha = .01$.

Incorrect analysis: We calculate $\overline{X}_B = 13.14$ and $\overline{X}_A = 15.14$, $s_A = 6.23$ and $s_B = 5.43$ so that the pooled estimate is $s_p = 5.84$ by Formula (9.8). The standardized difference between the two sample means under H_0 is $T_0 = -.64$ by Formula (9.9). This is not significant, even at the levels of .10 or .20, and the hypothesis that the population means are equal is therefore accepted.

Comment: The two *samples are not independent*, and the correct analysis is the one appropriate to paired samples (Section 9.3). To test the null hypothesis $H_0 : \mu(D) = 0$ against the alternative $H_L : \mu(D) < 0$, we calculate the sample average of differences, $\overline{D}$, and their standard deviation, $s(D)$, and standardize the mean, obtaining $T_0 = -3.74$. Since $-t_6(.01) = -3.14$, T_0 is significant at this level, and we reject the null hypothesis.

Example 17.3. (Two means)

Question: The average gain in weight of 17 rats, 9 fed on one experimental diet and 8 on another, was recorded and the usual calculations resulted in the following:

$$n_1 = 9 \qquad \overline{X}_1 = 50 \qquad s_1^2 = 108$$
$$n_2 = 8 \qquad \overline{X}_2 = 30 \qquad s_2^2 = 370$$

Are the two diets equally effective in increasing weight, or is the first one better? Take $\alpha = .01$.

Incorrect Analysis: The pooled estimate of the standard deviation is $s_p = 15.17$. Substituting in Formula (9.17), we obtain $T_0 = 2.71$. Since $t_{15}(.01) = 2.602$, we reject the hypothesis $H_0: \mu_1 - \mu_2 = 0$ and accept the alternative $H_R: \mu_1 - \mu_2 > 0$ at this level.

Comment: We *cannot assume* that the two *population variances* are *equal*, and therefore it makes no sense to estimate their "common value" by s_p^2. Instead, we use the statistic U_0 of Formula (9.10) which has a t distribution with degrees of freedom given by Formula (9.21). This formula yields $f = 11.78$, and we therefore take the degrees of freedom as 12. Since $t_{12}(.01) = 2.681$ and $U_0 = 2.62$, we accept H_0 at this level.

Example 17.4. (Prediction from a regression line)

Question: In a feeding experiment on 9 male rats, the Vitamin A intake (X) and weekly gain in weight (Y) were as follows:

X (units of Vitamin A)	Y (grams)
1.0	7
1.0	9
1.0	8
1.5	10
1.5	10
1.5	13
1.5	12
2.5	15
2.5	17

How many grams would a rat gain if given 5 units of the vitamin?

Partially-incorrect Analysis: By the methods of Sections 14.2 and 14.3, we find the equation of linear regression to be

$$\hat{\mu}(x) = 2.99 + 5.29x.$$

The line and the scatter diagram appear in Figure 17.1. From the diagram, the regression appears to be linear and this is supported by the analysis of variance (Section 14.3 b), from which we find that 87% of the total variation in Y is explained by its linear regression on X.

To predict the gain in weight for a particular rat given 5 units of the vitamin, we substitute 5 for x in the equation of the line and find the predicted gain in weight to be almost 30 grams. A 95% confidence interval for this predicted value is, by Formula (14.11),

$$29.44 \pm (2.365)(1.28)\sqrt{1 + 1/9 + 4.36}$$

or $\qquad 29.44 \pm 7.08.$

Comment : The analysis is correct up to the point where the line is to be used in predictions. Predicting growth corresponding to a value of X between 1 and 2.5 is meaningful, but we *cannot extrapolate from the line* to values outside this range. In other words, we have no right to assume that growth continues at the same rate indefinitely!

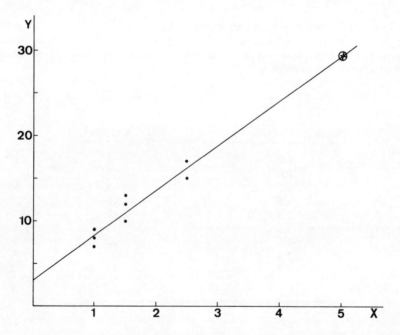

FIG. 17.1. Scatter diagram and regression line (Example 17.4)

Example 17.5.   (Linear regression)

Question: Is there a significant regression of Y on X in the following data? Test the hypothesis of no regression at the 5% level.

x	y
2	1
4	1
4	3
6	1.5
6	4.5
8	2
8	6

Incorrect Analysis: Since the average of Y seems to increase at a constant rate as X increases , we assume linear regression and calculate $S(x,x) = 29.71$, $S(x,y) = 14.86$, $S(y,y) = 21.93$, from which we get $b = .50$, $a = 0$ and $s = 1.70$. To test the null hypothesis $H_0 : \beta = 0$ against the right-sided alternative $H_R : \beta > 0$, we calculate T_0 from Formula (14.8) and compare it with $t_5(.05) = 2.015$. Since $T_0 = 1.6$, we accept H_0 and conclude that regression is not significant.

Comment: What went wrong? Clearly the average value of Y in this data increases as X increases (for a given x, $\hat{\mu}(x) = x/2$), and yet this is not reflected in the test of significance for the regression coefficient. The reason for this apparent contradiction can be seen from the scatter diagram in Figure 17.2 which shows Y increasing in variability as X increases. Therefore it cannot be assumed that the variance of Y at any fixed value of X is the same as at any other value (see (14.5), assumption (iii)). When the Y *variances are not homogeneous* for all values of X, the methods of Section 14.3 are not appropriate.

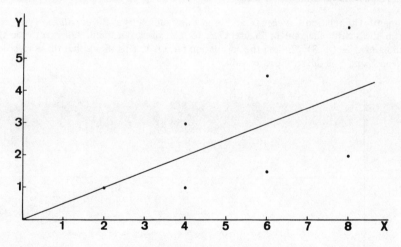

FIG. 17.2.   Scatter diagram (Example 17.5)

When the variances are heterogeneous and known, or known functions of X, a modification of the standard regression techniques, known as the method of *weighted regression,* can be used (see, for instance, Brownlee, 1960). Applying weighted regression to the above data, and using the estimate of the variance for each value of X as the reciprocal of the weight, we arrive at the linear regression equation $\hat{\mu}(x) = .50x$ (the same as before), but the value of the test statistic T_0 is now 3.27, and this is significant even at a lower level than 5%.

Example 17.6. (Regression)

Question: From the given data, would you conclude that X and Y were correlated?

x	y
7	8
6	4.5
5	2
4	0.5
3	0
2	0.5
1	2

Incorrect Analysis: We calculate the correlation coefficient r by Formula (14.13), using the preliminary results:

$n = 7$, $\Sigma x = 28$, $\Sigma x^2 = 140$, $\Sigma xy = 98$, $\Sigma y^2 = 92.75$, $\Sigma y = 17.50$. This yields $r = .76$, and $r^2 = .57$, which means that less than 60% of the variation in one of the variables is explained by the variation in the other.

Comment: The relation between Y and X in this example is of the *curvilinear* type, as is seen in the scatter diagram of Figure 17.3. In fact, the given points fall exactly on the parabola $\mu(x) = (x-3)^2/2$, and the correlation ratio is 1. This shows that the correlation between X and Y is the strongest possible.

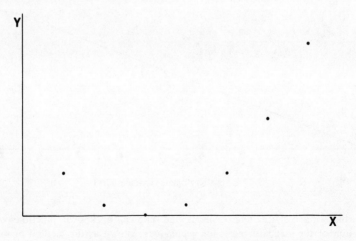

FIG. 17.3. Scatter diagram (Example 17.6)

Example 17.7.   (correlation)

Question: Y is a variable that can be observed at successively increasing levels of X, as in the following sample:

x	y
1	1
1	2
2	1
2	2
2	3
3	2
3	3

How strong is the correlation between X and Y?

Hasty Analysis: Using Formula (14.13), we find the coefficient of linear correlation r to be 0.50, so that $r^2 = .25$, which means that only one-quarter of the variation in Y is due to its regression on X.

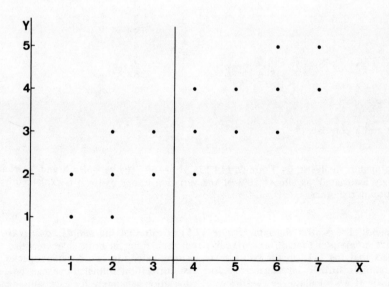

FIG. 17.4.   Truncated and complete scatter diagrams (Example 17.7)

Comment: If more data is collected (with X at levels higher than 3) a different picture might emerge. For instance, *the above sample may be only a portion* of a larger set of data that could have been collected if the experimenter had been more patient. The whole set is shown in the scatter diagram of Figure 17.4, and the set corresponding to X = 1, 2 or 3 is separated in the diagram from the other points by a vertical line showing the point of truncation in the observations. It is clear from the scatter diagram that, with the inclusion of more observations, a stronger relationship appears. In fact, if we calculate r^2 for the whole set of data, we get $r^2 = .67$, so that a full two-thirds of the variation in Y in this larger set can be attributed to X.

Example 17.8. (Correlation)

Question: The following table represents measurements of two characteristics, X and Y, in each of a sample of 13 cattle ticks.

x	y
1	1
1	2
1	3
2	1
2	2
2	3
3	1
3	2
3	3
5	5
5	6
6	5
6	6

Are X and Y correlated?

Questionable Analysis: By Formula (14.13), $r^2 = .69$. The variables X and Y are fairly strongly associated, as almost 70% of the variation in one of them is explained by the variation in the other.

Comment: The scatter diagram (Figure 17.5) reveals that the *sample consists of two distinct subsamples* that differ markedly from each other in both characteristics. This suggests that the ticks in the two subsamples may belong to two different species, and this requires further investigation before the correlation found above can be taken seriously. If we calculate the coefficient of correlation separately for each subsample, it turns out to be zero in both cases, which suggests that X and Y may not be associated at all!

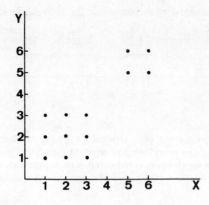

FIG. 17.5.   Scatter diagram (Example 17.8)

Example 17.9. (Equality of several means)

Question: Four observations were taken on each of 3 different treatments in a completely randomized design (Section 10.2) with the object of testing the hypothesis that the three population means are equal. The observations were as follows:

I	II	III
17	2	3
6	4	1
5	7	2
12	11	2

Should we accept this hypothesis at the 5% level?

Incorrect Analysis: By the methods of Section 10.3, we calculate the entries in the analysis of variance table and arrive at

Source of variation	Sum of squares	Degrees of freedom	Mean square
Between	128	2	64
Within	142	9	15.78
Total	270	11	

The variance ratio R is 4.06. Since $F_{2,9}$ (.05) = 4.26, R is not significant, and we accept the null hypothesis.

Comment: The means and standard deviations of the above three samples are as follows:

	I	II	III
$\overline{X} =$	10	6	2
$s^2 =$	31.33	15.33	0.67
$s \ =$	5.6	3.92	0.82

It appears that s is approximately proportional to $\overline{X}$, rather than being constant. The assumptions of the model are therefore not satisfied (see Section 10.2), and a *variance-stabilizing transformation* on the data is indicated. The appropriate transformation in this case is logarithmic (see Section 10.6), and the analysis of variance table after such a transformation becomes

Source of variation	Sum of squares	Degrees of freedom	Mean square
Between	.94	2	.47
Within	.61	9	.07
Total	1.55	11	

The variance ratio now is 6.93, which is significant at the 5% level. We thus reject the hypothesis of equality of the three population means.

Example 17.10. (Clinical trial)

Question: In a double-blind trial, 200 patients were administered a new drug and another 200 were given a placebo. Of the former, 10 succumbed to an infection, and of the latter 20. Is the drug effective in preventing the infection?

Incorrect Analysis: For each illness among the patients receiving the drug, there were two illnesses among the patients receiving the placebo. Therefore the drug reduces the probability of infection by a half.

Comment: The above analysis *ignores important information,* namely the number of patients who were free from infection from the two groups. Taking this into account, we set up the 2 x 2 table:

	Infection	No Infection
Drug	10	190
Placebo	20	180

and calculate the statistic Y (Formula (12.6)). The result is $Y = 2.92$. Since this is smaller than $\chi_1^2(.05) = 3.84$, we conclude at the 5% level that there is no association between the two variables of classification and hence that the drug is no more and no less effective in preventing infection than the placebo.

Example 17.11. (The P–value)

Question: Paired samples were taken to test the hypothesis of equality of two population means against the alternative that they are not equal, and resulted in: $\bar{D} = 15$, $s(D) = 30$, $n = 16$. What is the P–value of the test statistic?

Incorrect calculation: Under the hypothesis tested, the standardized $\bar{D}$ has a t–distribution with 15 degrees of freedom. Therefore the P–value of $\bar{D}$ is $P(\bar{D} \geqslant 15)$, which is

$$P(T \geqslant \frac{15 - 0}{30/\sqrt{16}}) = P(T \geqslant 2).$$

From the t–tables with 15 degrees of freedom, this is equal to .032.

Comment: The P–value is the probability of observing the value of the test statistic or a more extreme value. Since the alternative hypothesis is two-sided, the significant values of T_0 are *in the two tails of the t-distribution*, and therefore the P-value of $\bar{D}$ is $P(|T| \geqslant 2)$. By symmetry of the t-distribution, this is twice the value calculated above, i.e. 064.

Right-Sided Alternative   **Two-Sided Alternative**

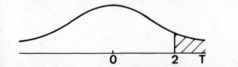
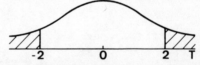

FIG. 17.6. Calculating the P-value corresponding to $T_0 = 2$ (Example 17.11)

Example 17.12. (The null hypothesis)

Question: Data from two independent samples yielded the following:

$$n_1 = 10, \qquad n_2 = 8, \qquad s_1^2/s_2^2 = 4.$$

What conclusion can we draw about the null hypothesis if
$H_0: \sigma_1^2 = \sigma_2^2$ is tested against $H_R: \sigma_1^2 > \sigma_2^2$?

Incorrect interpretation: Using the notation of Section 11.2, we compare $F_0 = 4$ with the percentile $F_{9,7}(.05) = 3.68$. Since F_0 is larger than 3.68, the probability that H_0 is true is less than 5%.

Comment: Comparing the variance ratio F_0 with a percentile of the F–distribution makes sense only if H_0 is true, because it is under this assumption that F_0 has an F–distribution with 9 and 7 degrees of freedom. The correct conclusion is: If H_0 is true, $P(F_0 \geqslant 4)$ is less than 5% , and therefore H_0 is rejected at the 5% level.

REFERENCE

Brownlee, K.A. (1960). *Statistical Theory and Methodology in Science and Engineering.* Wiley, New York.

CHAPTER 18
Computer Programs

18.1. INTRODUCTION

Over the past two decades, computers have established themselves as essential tools for scientific investigations. With the introduction of high-level programming languages like FORTRAN, BASIC, ALGOL and others, computers have become more readily adaptable to the needs of an individual. At the same time, the rapid development of microprocessor technology has led to the availability of desk-top microcomputers and sophisticated programmable calculators for personal use. Most microcomputers are manufactured for programming in BASIC, although some of them can be programmed in other high-level languages.

This chapter contains twenty-seven short programs written in (CP/M)BASIC.They can readily be used in any computer system, including personal microcomputers, and may be adapted to programmable calculators after appropriate modification. Each program is listed and illustrated independently of the others.

The reader is encouraged to use a desk-top microcomputer for the bulk of the statistical computations required in data analysis. The programs given in this chapter are easy to apply to one's own data; at the same time, they are meant to assist those readers who are not already familiar with the techniques of BASIC programming in acquiring a working knowledge of this computer language. For multiple regression outputs and other sophisticated data processing, a high-speed digital computer is needed, and the task may then be performed with the aid of a statistical package (such as BMD, SPSS, PSTAT, MINITAB, etc.) available at the user's computer center.

A *computer program* (soft ware) is a finite set of statements which instructs the computer to perform a certain task. Although it is possible to write a computer program in machine language where instructions use only the two symbols 0 and 1, programming in machine language is technical, time-consuming and requires high precision. In order to facilitate programming, various high-level languages such FORTRAN, ALGOL, COBOL and BASIC have been developed. These languages use English words and phrases to represent steps in the program sequence and use mathematical symbols to express mathematical operations for computation. Statements such as "READ", "PRINT", "GOTO", "IF A $<$ B THEN X $= \emptyset$" are typical. These simple statements, when included in a program sequence, call for complex computer operations and have to be translated by a machine code program called a *compiler* (which is stored in the computer) so as to enable the computer to execute the program.

18.2. PROGRAMS IN BASIC

The BASIC (*B*eginner's *A*ll-Purpose *S*ymbolic *I*nstruction *C*ode) is an interactive programming language developed in 1963 at Dartmouth College (U.S.A.) by Kemeny and Kurtz. This language has been found suitable for beginners to learn yet powerful enough to carry out considerably complex computations. There are many variations of the programming language BASIC, depending upon the microcomputer system in use. Extended BASIC offers additional facilities for writting sophisticated programs and has better string handling capability*. Before using a microcomputer it is advisable to learn the form of BASIC used by the machine and the commands necessary to print the program and obtain the printed output through the printer after execution.

A BASIC program consists of one or more statements typed on a keyboard. If the statement is preceded by an integer sequence lying in the range 1 to 9999, it is saved as part of a program which may be executed in whole or in part later. Such statements may be erased or modified even after they are saved. An unnumbered statement is executed as soon as its completion is signified by a carriage return on the input keyboard.

Readers unfamiliar with the computer language may find the following summary of some commonly used BASIC commands helpful.

18.2a. Input/Output Commands

READ : It instructs the computer to refer to a DATA statement and read the corresponding entries in it. For example,

        10 READ X, Y, Z
        100 DATA 10, 20.9, 11.6

indicates that $X = 10, Y = 20.9, Z = 11.6$.

INPUT : This command instructs the computer to obtain the data directly from the user. At this stage in the program, a question mark (or a string, if provided) appears on the terminal, and the user is then expected to type in the data. For example,

        25 INPUT X, Y

indicates that values of X and Y are to be provided in that order. Since it calls for those values during the execution of the program, an INPUT statement does not require a DATA statement.

PRINT : It prints text and data and also evaluates expressions and variables before printing. The statement takes one of the following general forms:-

---

* Our programs in this chapter will not use string manipulation, for the sake of simplicity.

```
50 PRINT  expression, expression,..
60 PRINT  "symbols", "symbols",..
70 PRINT  "symbols", "expressions".
```

In some microcomputers PRINT is also used to skip one line and format the output data. In that case, the general form is:-

(Line number) PRINT

In CPM BASIC run on the PCC 2000 microcomputer, the following statement is used to skip a line:-

(Line number) PRINT

In the system we have used, PRINT is replaced by LPRINT for actual printing of text or data by means of the printer interfaced to the PCC 2000. These statements may need modification for other microcomputer systems.

18.2b. Specification and Documentation Commands

DIM: This command reserves spaces for subscripted variables. The DIM (Dimension) command, if used, must be the first statement in a BASIC program. It is acceptable to overdimension (that is, to povide more than the necessary space) for a subscripted variable, but not to underdimension. For example,

```
10 DIM  X(20), Y(15), Z(29)
```

indicates that 20, 15, and 29 locations are reserved, respectively, for X, Y, and Z.

DATA : This statement contains data (numerical or string) for variables listed in a READ statement. The DATA statement may appear anywhere in a BASIC program except on the last line (which is reserved for the END statement) or the first line if a DIM statement is used. A DATA statement takes the general form:-

(Line number) DATA data value, data value, ..

REM : This is used to include remarks within the program. Any number of remarks may be included to explain the nature and purpose of the program and identify important parts of it. It is a nonexecutable statement. The following example illustrates its use:-

```
10 REM  THIS PROGRAM ARRANGES DATA
20 REM  IN INCREASING ORDER
```

RESTORE : This command resets the "data pointer" to the beginning of the first DATA statement in the program. Thus, after a set of data has been used, RESTORE makes it available for reuse in the same program. It takes the general form:-

(Line number) RESTORE

18.2c. Loop and Subroutine Commands

FOR-NEXT : This combination is used for setting up a "loop" to execute the statements placed between the FOR command and the NEXT command a specified number of times. Unless otherwise stated, the loop variable is incremented by $+ 1$ at each step. For example,

```
10  FOR I = 1  to  11  STEP  2
20  . . . .
30  . . . .
40  NEXT  I
```

indicates that statements 20 and 30 are to be executed for $I = 1, 3, 5, 7, 9,$ and 11.

GOSUB-RETURN : The GOSUB statement directs the processing sequence to a subroutine (a self-contained sequence of operations). The RETURN statement returns the processing sequence to the statement immediately following the most recently executed GOSUB command. For example,

```
 10  . . .
 15  GOSUB  40
 20  . . .
 25  GOSUB  40
 30  . . .
 40  . . .
 50  . . .
 60  RETURN
 70 . . .
100  END
```

indicates that statements 40 and 50 are to be executed after 10; following that, the computer returns to statement 20 for execution,then goes to 40 and 50 before returning to statement 30.

18.2d. Logic Commands

GOTO   :   This is an unconditional branching command which transfers control to a specified line number. For example:

```
50  GOTO  10
```

instructs the computer to proceed to statement 10 for the continuation of the processing sequence.

IF-THEN : This is a conditional branching command. If the expression following IF is true, the processing sequence is transferred to a specified line number. For example,

```
25  IF  A ≤ B  THEN  50
```

indicates that control is transferred to statement 50 if A ≤ B
following 25 is executed.

STOP : This is used to stop the execution of a program before
reached. It has the general form:-

(Line number) STOP

END : This is always the last statement of the program and has the form

(Line number) END

18.2e. Arithmetic Commands

DEF : The DEF (Definition) command allows the user to define frequently used one-line functions in a program. For example,

10 DEF FN P(X) = X*X + X

indicates that henceforth P(X) will stand for the function $X^2 + X$.

LET : This is an optional assignment statement used for computation or for manipulation of an arithmetic variable. It is used to compute and store the numerical   value of the variable. For example,

10 LET X = 1
20 LET Y = 2*X*X + X−3

indicates that X is given the value 1 and $Y = 2X^2 + X−3$ becomes zero as soon as statement 20 is executed.

18.2f. Operating Commands

Commands such as LOAD, SAVE, RUN, COPY, LIST, DELETE, RESET are essential for the operation and development of programs. Every computer has its own operating system which describes exact formats for the above commands.

BASIC ignores spaces. "READ A, B" may equally well appear as "R E A D A, B". However, proper use of conventional spacing contributes to better clarity in the reading of a program. One should also be aware of the potential ambiguity in reading printed text that contains either the alphabet letter "O" or the numeric symbol "∅" (zero).

Arithmetical and Relational Symbols

+	addition
−	subtraction
*	multiplication
/	division
↑	raise to a power
=	is equal to
>	is greater than
<	is less than
> = or = >	is greater than or equal to
< = or = <	is less than or equal to
< > or > <	is not equal to

BASIC requires that an arithmetic formula be contained in one line, with no subscripts or "double-decker" functions.

18.2h. Intrinsic Functions

An intrinsic function is one whose meaning has been incorporated in the BASIC compiler. The following expressions are some intrinsic functions which can be evaluated when a value is assigned to the argument:

SIN(X)	calculates the sine of X radians
COS(X)	calculates the cosine of X radians
TAN(X)	calculates the tangent of X radians
ABS(Y)	calculates the absolute value of Y
SQR(Y)	calculates the square root of Y
EXP(Y)	calculates the exponential function e^Y
LOG(Y)	calculates the natural logarithm of Y
INT(R)	calculates the largest integer less than or equal to R
SGN(R)	equals $+1$ if $R > 0$, equals 0 if $R = 0$, equals -1 if $R < 0$

18.2i. Representation of Variables

In BASIC, variables can be represented by a letter (X), a letter followed by a digit (Y4), or either of the above followed by the symbol $ (X$ or Y4$). Representations ending with $ are usually assigned to "string variables" or alphanumeric data (data which contains letters of the alphabet, digits from 0 to 9, and other symbols available on the keyboard). Representations without the $ sign are usually restricted to numerical variables. Subscripted variables are used for lists and tables; the subscript may be an integer (as in X(10)), a variable (as in P(I)), or an arithmetic statement (as in L(2 + K)). For subscripted variables, it is necessary to reserve sufficient storage space in the computer's memory by means of the DIM statement mentioned earlier.

18.3. LIST OF PROGRAMS

230

Program CHIS1

(Text reference: §12.1, page 144)

Description: This program calculates Chi-square for
the comparison of two proportions in a 2x2 table.

Formula used:

$$\text{Chi-square } X2 = \frac{(AD-BC)^2 (A+B+C+D)}{(A+B)(C+D)(A+C)(B+D)}$$

where A,B,C,D are the observed frequencies in the four
cells of the table

A	B
C	D

Data entry: Data lines are from 100 to 199 and the data
can be entered as follows:

        100   DATA A,B,C,D

Program:

```
5   LPRINT"CHI-SQUARE CALCULATION"
10  LPRINT"FOR 2 BY 2 TABLES"
11  LPRINT"**********************"
12  LPRINT""
15  LPRINT""
20  LPRINT""
25  READ A,B,C,D
30  LET S=A+B+C+D
35  LET M=(A*D)-(B*C)
40  LET L=(A+B)*(C+D)*(B+D)*(A+C)
45  LET X=(M*M*S)/L
50  DEF FN R(I) = INT (I*100! +.5)/100!
55  LPRINT" DATA WERE ";A;B
60  LPRINT""
65  LPRINT"               ";C;D
70  LPRINT""
75  LPRINT""
80  LPRINT"CHI-SQUARE X2 = ";FN R(X)
85  LPRINT""
90  LPRINT""
95  GOTO 15
200 END
```

Illustration: To calculate the Chi-square statistic for
   the data of Example 12.1 (page 144) perform the
   following:

```
LOAD "CHIS1"
100  DATA  16, 9, 7, 14
LIST
RUN
```

Printout:

```
CHI-SQUARE CALCULATION
FOR 2 BY 2 TABLES
**********************


 DATA WERE  16   9

            7   14


CHI-SQUARE X2 =   4. 29
```

Program CHIS2

(Text reference: §12.1, page 143)

Description: This program calculates Chi-square with
  Yates' continuity correction in a 2x2 table.

Formula used:

$$\text{Chi-square } X2 = \frac{[\,|AD-BC| \; - \; \frac{1}{2}(A+B+C+D)\,]^2\,[A+B+C+D]}{(A+B)\,(C+D)\,(A+C)\,(B+D)}$$

where A,B,C,D are the observed frequencies in the four
cells of the table

A	B
C	D

Data entry: Data lines are from 120 to 199 and data
  are entered as

        120   DATA   A,B,C,D

Program:

```
10 LPRINT"CHI-SQUARE CALCULATION"
15 LPRINT" WITH CONTINUITY CORRECTION"
20 LPRINT"(2 BY 2 CONTINGENCY TABLE"
25 LPRINT"*************************"
30 LPRINT""
35 READ A,B,C,D
40 LET S=A+B+C+D
42 LET M=ABS((A*D)-(B*C))
45 LET L=(A+B)*(C+D)*(B+D)*(A+C)
50 LET N=(M-(1/2)*S)*(M-(1/2)*S)*S
55 DEF FN R(I)= INT(I*100!+.5)/100!
60 LPRINT" DATA WERE ";A;B
65 LPRINT""
70 LPRINT"               ";C;D
75 LPRINT""
85 LPRINT" CHI-SQUARE X2 = "; FN R(N/L)
90 LPRINT""
95 LPRINT""
115 GOTO 35
200 END
```

Remark: Line 55 of the program can also be entered
  on the keyboard as

    55 DEF FN R(I) = INT (I*E2 + .5)/E2

Illustration: To calculate the Chi-square statistic
  with Yates' correction for the data of Example 12.1
  (page 144), perform the following:

```
LOAD "CHIS2"
120  DATA  16, 9, 7, 14
LIST
RUN
```


Printout:

```
CHI-SQUARE CALCULATION
 WITH CONTINUITY CORRECTION
(2 BY 2 CONTINGENCY TABLE
***************************

DATA WERE   16   9

            7   14

CHI-SQUARE X2 =   3.15
```

Program CHIS3

(Text references: §13.1 and § 13.2, pages 151,155)

Description: This program calculates the Chi-square statistic for a contingency table, Pearson's coefficient of contingency and Cramér's coefficient.

Formulas used:

(i)   Chi-square $Y = \sum_{I=1}^{M} \sum_{J=1}^{N} \frac{[O(I,J)-E(I,J)]^2}{E(I,J)}$

where

M = number of rows,

N = number of columns,

O(I,J) = observed frequency entered at row I and column J,

E(I,J) = Expected frequency corresponding to O(I,J), calculated as
E(I,J) = R(I).C(J)/S1

with

$R(I) = \sum_{J=1}^{N} O(I,J)$, $C(J) = \sum_{I=1}^{M} O(I,J)$,

S1 = sum of all the observed frequencies O(I,J).

(ii) Pearson's coefficient of contingency

$P = [Y/(Y+S1)]^{\frac{1}{2}}$

(iii) Cramér's coefficient

$C = [Y/(S1.\min(M-1,N-1))]^{\frac{1}{2}}$

Data entry: Data lines are from 211 to 299 and the data should be entered as

230   DATA M,N

235   DATA ENTRIES IN ROW 1 TO ROW M

For example the following 3x3 contingency table is
entered as

20	32	18
18	20	12
12	8	10

```
230  DATA  3, 3
235  DATA  20, 32, 18, 18, 20, 12, 12, 8, 10
```

Program:

```
10 LPRINT"CHI-SQUARE CALCULATION FOR LARGER TABLES"
15 LPRINT" PEARSONS AND CRAMERS COEFFICIENTS"
16 LPRINT"*********************************************"
17 LPRINT""
20 DIM X(25,25)
25 READ M,N
30 LET S1=0
35 FOR I=1 TO M
40 FOR J=1 TO N
45 LET R(I)=0
50 LET C(J)=0
55 NEXT J
60 NEXT I
65 FOR I=1 TO M
70 FOR J=1 TO N
75 READ X(I,J)
80 LET R(I)=R(I)+X(I,J)
85 LET C(J)=C(J)+X(I,J)
90 NEXT J
95 LET S1=S1+R(I)
100 NEXT I
105 LET C=0
110 FOR I=1 TO M
115 FOR J=1 TO N
120 LET E=R(I)*C(J)/S1
125 LET C=C+(X(I,J)-E)^2/E
130 LPRINT X(I,J),
135 NEXT J
140 LPRINT""
145 NEXT I
150 LPRINT""
155 LET Y=INT(C*1000!+.5)/1000!
160 LPRINT"CHI-SQUARE      =";Y
165 LPRINT"DEGREES OF FREEDOM ";(M-1) * (N-1)
170 LPRINT""
```

18.3. CHIS3

```
175 IF M<N THEN L=M-1 ELSE L=N-1
185 LET P=SQR(Y/(Y+S1))
190 LET C=SQR(Y/(S1*L))
195 LPRINT"PEARSONS COEFF. =";P
200 LPRINT"CRAMERS COEFF. =";C
205 LPRINT""
210 GOTO 25
300 END
```

Illustration: For Example 13.1 (page 155), perform the following:

```
        LOAD "CHIS3"
        230   DATA  3,3
        235   DATA  30, 15, 19, 17, 6, 6, 27, 8, 16
        LIST
        RUN
```

Printout:

```
CHI-SQUARE CALCULATION FOR LARGER TABLES
  PEARSONS AND CRAMERS COEFFICIENTS
************************************

  30              15             19
  17              6              6
  27              8              16

CHI-SQUARE      = 2.226
DEGREES OF FREEDOM  4

PEARSONS COEFF. = .123382
CRAMERS COEFF.  = .0879157
```

Program DESC1

(Text reference: §8.2b, page 95)

Description: This program arranges numerical data in
    ascending order.

Data Entry: Data lines are from 121 to 199. We enter
    data as

       Line number   DATA   N, X, Y, Z, ...

    where N is the number of data points and X, Y, Z, ...
    are the data points to be sorted out.

Program:


```
10 LPRINT" PROGRAM SORTS OUT DATA IN ASCENDING ORDER"
20 DIM X(100)
25 LPRINT""
30 READ N
35 FOR C=1 TO N
40 READ X(C)
45 NEXT C
50 FOR C=1 TO N-1
55 FOR I=1 TO N-C
60 LET P=X(I)
65 LET Q=X(I+1)
70 IF P<=Q THEN 85
75 LET X(I)=Q
80 LET X(I+1)=P
85 NEXT I
90 NEXT C
95 FOR C=1 TO N
100 LPRINT   X(C);
105 LPRINT ",";
110 NEXT C
115 LPRINT""
120 LPRINT""
200 GOTO 30
210 END
```


Illustration: Arrange the following two discrete data
    sets in ascending order:

        (i)   1, 101, 35, 78, 6
        (ii)   10.5, 9.8, 105, 71.9, 32.8, 61.7

Perform the following:

```
LOAD "DESC1"
125   DATA   5, 1, 101, 35, 78, 6
130   DATA   6, 10.5, 9.8, 105, 71.9, 32.8, 61.7
LIST
RUN
```

Printout:

PROGRAM SORTS OUT DATA IN ASCENDING ORDER
****

1 , 6 , 35 , 78 , 101 ,

9.8 , 10.5 , 32.8 , 61.7 , 71.9 , 105 ,

Remark: Once discrete data is arranged in increasing
         order we can calculate the median, range etc.
         immediately. For example, for (i) the median is
         35 and for (ii) it is (32.8 + 61.7)/2 = 47.25.

Program DESC2

(Text reference: §7.2a, 8.2a, pages 86, 94)

Description: This program computes: the mean, standard
  deviation, variance, coefficient of variation and standard error of the mean from a set of raw data.

Formulas used:

   (i)   Mean: $M = \Sigma X / N$

   (ii)   Variance: $V = [\Sigma X^2 - \frac{(\Sigma X)^2}{N}] / (N-1)$

   (iii)   Standard deviation: $D = \sqrt{V}$

   (iv)   Coefficient of variation: $C = \frac{D}{M} \times 100\%$

   (v)   Standard error of mean: $E = D / \sqrt{N}$

  where X is the value of an individual observation and
  N is the number of observations.

Data Entry: Data lines are from 121 to 199. Data is
  entered as

        150   DATA   N, X(1), X(2), ..., X(N)

  where X(1), X(2), ..., X(N) are the N observations.

Program:

```
5   DIM X(100)
10 LPRINT"COMPUTATION OF MEAN, VARIANCE,STD. DEVIATION"
15 LPRINT"COEF. OF VARIATION AND STD. ERROR OF MEAN"
16 LPRINT"*************************************************"
17 LPRINT""
20 LET S=0
25 LET S2=0
30 READ N
35 FOR I=1 TO N
40 READ X(I)
45 LET S=S+X(I)
50 LET S2=S2+X(I)^2
55 NEXT I
60 LET M=S/N
65 LET V=(S2 - (S*S) / N)/(N-1)
70 LET D=SQR(V)
75 LET C=(D/M) /100
80 LET E=D / SQR(N)
```

```
85 LPRINT "NO OF OBSERVATIONS       ";N
90 LPRINT "MEAN                     ";M
95 LPRINT "STD. DEVIATION           ";D
100 LPRINT"VARIANCE                 ";V
105 LPRINT"COEF. VARIATION          ";C
110 LPRINT"STD. ERROR OF MEAN       ";E
115 LPRINT""
120 LPRINT""
200 GOTO 20
210 END
```

Illustration: Calculate the Mean,Variance,Standard
   deviation,Coefficient of variation and Standard
   error of the mean of the data of Example 7.1 (page 87).

Perform the following:

```
LOAD "DESC2"
150 DATA 51,68,60,48,84,88,68,76,52,52,64,60,64
151 DATA 56,52,72,60,48,40,52,64,100,52,64,48,68
152 DATA 76,80,92,56,96,85,88,40,60,52,84,76,64
153 DATA 92,44,36,44,92,48,48,52,68,72,28,56,32
LIST
RUN
```

Printout:

```
COMPUTATION OF MEAN, VARIANCE,STD.DEVIATION
COEF. OF VARIATION AND STD. ERROR OF MEAN
*************************************************

NO OF OBSERVATIONS        51
MEAN                      63.1569
STD. DEVIATION            17.6118
VARIANCE                  310.175
COEF. VARIATION           2.78858E-03
STD. ERROR OF MEAN        2.46614
```

Program DESC3

(Text reference:§7.2b,8.2a, pages 88,94)

Description: This program computes: the mean, median,
   variance and standard deviation from a set of observations grouped into class intervals of equal width.

Formulas used:

Sum of frequencies: $C(N) = \Sigma_{i=1}^{N} F(I)$.

   Mean: $M = (\Sigma_{I=1}^{N} F(I)X(I))/C(N)$

   Variance:

$$V = \frac{\Sigma_{I=1}^{N} X(I)^2 F(I) - (\Sigma_{I=1}^{N} X(I)F(I))^2/C(N)}{C(N)-1}$$

   Standard deviation: $S = \sqrt{V}$

   Median: $M1 = B + D.W/F$

   where
      N = Number of class intervals, $N \leq 20$,
         X(I) = Midpoint of the Ith class interval
         $(I = 1,2,...,N)$,
      F(I) = Frequency in the Ith class interval,
      B   = Lower limit of the class containing
             the median,
      W   = Width of the class intervals,
      Fl   = Cumulative frequency up to B,
      D   = (C(N)/2) - Fl,
      F   = Frequency of the class containing the median.

Data entry: Data lines are from 311 to 409. Data is
   entered as

      320   DATA N, F(1), X(1), F(2), X(2),..., F(N), X(N)

Program:

```
10 LPRINT"DESCRIPTIVE STATISTICS FOR GROUPED DATA"
11 LPRINT"*******************************************"
12 LPRINT""
14 LPRINT""
30 READ N
40 LET S1=0
50 LET S2=0
60 LET C(0)=0
70 FOR I=1 TO N
```

```
80 READ F(I),X(I)
90 LET S1 = S1 + F(I)*X(I)
100 LET S2=S2+F(I)*X(I)*X(I)
110 LET C(I) =C(I-1)+F(I)
120 NEXT I
130 LET M=S1/C(N)
140 LET V=(S2-(S1*S1/C(N)))/C(N)
150 LET S=SQR(V)
160 FOR I=1 TO N
170 IF C(I) > C(N)/2 THEN 190
180 NEXT I
190 LET W=X(2)-X(1)
200 LET B= X(I)-W/2
220 LET D= (C(N)/2)-C(I-1)
230 LET M1=B+D*W/F(I)
240 LPRINT"MEAN                        =";M
241 LPRINT""
242 LPRINT""
250 LPRINT"VARIANCE                    =";V
251 LPRINT""
252 LPRINT""
260 LPRINT"STANDARD DEVIATION     =";S
261 LPRINT""
262 LPRINT""
270 LPRINT"MEDIAN                      =";M1
310 GOTO 30
410 END
```

Illustration: Find the mean, median, variance and standard
  deviation of the sample data of Example 7.2 (page 88).
  We have to input the number of classes, midpoint of
  class intervals and class frequencies as data in the
  above program. Perform the following:

```
    LOAD "DESC2"
    320   DATA  9, 1, 25, 3, 35, 8, 45, 10, 55, 13, 65,
                5, 75, 6, 85, 4, 95, 1, 105
    LIST
    RUN
```

Printout:

```
DESCRIPTIVE STATISTICS FOR GROUPED DATA
*******************************************

MEAN                    = 63.8235

VARIANCE                = 324.106

STANDARD DEVIATION      = 18.003

MEDIAN                  = 62.6923
```

Program DEVS1

(Text reference: §11.2, page 136)

Description: This program compares the standard
  deviations of two populations by means of
  confidence intervals and hypothesis testing.

Formulas used:

(i)   A confidence interval for σ_1^2/σ_2^2 at
       level $(1-\alpha)$: R1 $\leq \sigma_1^2/\sigma_2^2 \leq$ R2

where

        R1 = R/F1

        R2 = R.F2

        F1 = $F_{N1-1,N2-1}(\alpha/2)$

        F2 = $F_{N2-1,N1-1}(\alpha/2)$

        N1 = size of the sample drawn from the first
             population
        N2 = size of the sample drawn from the second
             population

(ii)   In testing the null hypothesis H_0: $\sigma_1^2/\sigma_2^2 = k$
       against two-sided alternatives, H_0 is
       rejected at significance level α if

        R - kF1 > 0 or R - kF2 < 0

otherwise H_0 is accepted.

In testing the same null hypothesis against H_R: $\sigma_1^2/\sigma_2^2 > k$
at significance level α, H_0 is rejected if
R - kF3 > 0 where F3 = $F_{N1-1,N2-1}(\alpha)$.

(Note that σ_1 is the standard deviation suspected of
being larger than σ_2).

Data entry: Data lines are from 221 to 349 and the
  data is entered as

        300 DATA D, N1, N2, S1, S2
where D is a dummy variable with

        D = 0 when no test of hypothesis is needed,
        D = 1 when testing against two sided alternatives,
        D = 2 when testing against one-sided alternatives.

If a hypothesis is to be tested, the hypothesized value k, of σ_1^2/σ_2^2 is entered as an INPUT during program execution.

F percentiles corresponding to specified values of α are also entered as INPUT during program execution.

Program:

```
10 LPRINT"PROGRAM COMPARS TWO STANDARD DEVIATIONS"
15 LPRINT"OBTAINS CONFIDENCE INTERVALS"
16 LPRINT"TESTS HYPOTHESES"
20 LPRINT"*******************************"
25 LPRINT""
30 LPRINT""
35 READ D,N1,N2,S1,S2
40 LET R=(S1*S1)/(S2*S2)
45 LPRINT"ENTER F1=F(ALPHA/2) FOR"N1-1","N2-1"DEG. FREEDOM"
50 INPUT F1
55 LET R1=R/F1
60 LPRINT"ENTER F2=F(ALPHA/2)FOR"N2-1","N1-1;"DEG. FREEDOM"
65 INPUT F2
70 LET R2=R*F2
75 LPRINT"          F1=";F1
80 LPRINT"          F2=";F2
85 LPRINT""
90 LPRINT"THE CONFIDENCE INTERVAL IS :"
95 LPRINT R1;"TO";R2 "INCLUDING END POINTS"
100 LPRINT""
105 IF D=0 THEN 35
110 LPRINT"ENTER K=HYPOTHESIZED RATIO OF SIGMAS"
115 INPUT K
120 LPRINT"          K=";K
125 IF D=1 THEN 185
130 LPRINT"ENTER F3=F(ALPHA) FOR"N1-1","N2-1"DEG FREEDOM"
135 INPUT F3
140 LPRINT"          F3=";F3
145 LPRINT""
150 LPRINT""
155 IF R-K*F3>0 THEN 175
160 LPRINT"ACCEPT NULL HYPOTHESIS FOR ONE TAIL TEST"
165 LPRINT""
170 GOTO 35
175 LPRINT"REJECT NULL HYPOTHESIS FOR ONE TAIL TEST"
180 LPRINT""
181 GOTO 35
185 IF R-K*F1>0 THEN 210
190 IF R-K/F2<0 THEN 210
195 LPRINT"ACCEPT NULL HYPOTHESIS FOR TWO TAIL TEST"
```

```
200 LPRINT""
205 GOTO 35
210 LPRINT"REJECT NULL HYPOTHESIS FOR TWO TAIL TEST"
215 LPRINT""
220 GOTO 35
350 END
```

Illustration. In Example 11.1 (page 137) the hypothesis
to be tested is

$$H_0: \sigma_1^2/\sigma_2^2 = 1 \text{ against } H_A: \sigma_1^2/\sigma_2^2 > 1 \text{ at level } \alpha = 5\%.$$

Here Nl = 14, N = 7. Perform the following

```
LOAD "DEVS1"
250  DATA  2, 14, 7, 13.75, 10.41
LIST
RUN
```

When asked for INPUT during program execution enter
$F_{13,6}(.05) = 3.98, F_{6,13}(.05) = 2.92$, k = 1 and

$F_{13,6}(.05) = 3.98$, in this order.

Printout:

```
PROGRAM COMPARS TWO STANDARD DEVIATIONS
OBTAINS CONFIDENCE INTERVALS
TESTS HYPOTHESES
*********************************


ENTER F1=F(ALPHA/2) FOR 13 , 6 DEG. FREEDOM


ENTER F2=F(ALPHA/2) FOR 6 , 13 DEG. FREEDOM
      F1= 3.98
      F2= 2.92

THE CONFIDENCE INTERVAL IS :
   .43835 TO 5.09433 INCLUDING END POINTS

ENTER K=HYPOTHESIZED RATIO OF SIGMAS
      K= 1
ENTER F3=F(ALPHA) FOR 13 , 6 DEG. FREEDOM
      F3= 3.98


ACCEPT NULL HYPOTHESIS FOR ONE TAIL TEST
```

Program DEVS2

(Text reference: §11.3, page 138)

Description: This program tests the hypothesis that
  the standard deviations of K normal populations are
  equal (K > 2) by using Bartlett's test.

Formula used: Let the sample N(I) have variance

$$V(I), \ I = 1,2,\ldots, \ K \ (K > 2).$$

Let $S1 = \Sigma_{I=1}^{K} (N(I)-1)$

$\quad S2 = \Sigma_{I=1}^{K} \ \dfrac{1}{N(I) \ - \ 1}$

$\quad S3 = \Sigma_{I=1}^{K} \ (N(I)-1)V(I)$

$\quad S4 = \Sigma_{I=1}^{K} \ (N(I)-1)LOG(V(I))/LOG(10)$

$\quad S5 = S3/S1$

$\quad M = 2.3026 \ \{(S1)(LOG(S5)/LOG(10))-S4\}$

$\quad C = 1 + [S2 - 1/S1]/3(K-1).$

The test statistic is A = M/C, and the null hypothesis
is rejected if

$$A > \chi_{k-1}^{2}(\alpha)$$

where $\chi_{k-1}^{2}(\alpha)$ is $100(1-\alpha)$ percentile of the chi-square
distribution with (K-1) degrees of freedom.

The χ^2 value is to be provided as INPUT during program
execution.

Data entry: Data lines are from 220 to 299 and enter
  data as

        260   DATA K, N(1), S(1), N(2), S(2), ...,
                    N(K), S(K)

Program:

```
10 LPRINT"COMPARISON OF SEVERAL STANDARD DEVIATIONS"
11 LPRINT"*********************************************"
15 LPRINT""
20 LPRINT""
25 DIM N(20),V(20)
30 READ K
35 LET S1=0
40 LET S2=0
45 LET S3=0
50 LET S4=0
55 FOR I=1 TO K
60 READ N(I),V(I)
65 LET N1=N(I)-1
70 LET S1=S1+N1
75 LET N2=1/(N(I)-1)
80 LET S2=S2+N2
85 LET N3=(N(I)-1)*V(I)
90 LET S3=S3+N3
95 LET N4=(N(I)-1)*LOG(V(I))/LOG(10)
100 LET S4=S4+N4
105 NEXT I
110 LET S5=S3/S1
115 LET M=(2.3026)*(S1 *LOG(S5)/LOG(10)-S4)
120 LPRINT"M=";M
125 LPRINT""
130 LET C=1+((S2 - (1/S1))/(3*(K-1)))
135 LPRINT"C=";C
140 LET A=M/C
145 LPRINT""
155 LPRINT" THE TEST STATISTIC M/C=";A
160 LPRINT""
165 LPRINT"ENTER CHI-SQ. X2 FOR"K-1"DEG. FREEDOM"
170 LPRINT""
175 INPUT X2
177 LPRINT"CHISQUARE VALUE=";X2
180 IF A-X2 > 0 THEN 210
185 LPRINT " A-X2=";A-X2
190 LPRINT""
200 LPRINT" ACCEPT NULL HYPOTHESIS"
205 GOTO 30
210 LPRINT" REJECT NULL HYPOTHESIS"
215 GOTO 30
300 END
```

Illustration: In Example 11.2 (page 139), K = 8,
   N(I) = 11 for I = 1, 2, ..., 8, α = .05 and
   $\chi_7^2(.05)$ = 14.07.   Perform the following:

```
     LOAD "DEVS2"
     250   DATA   8, 11, 80124, 11, 787882, 11, 534183,
                  11, 458031, 11, 348772, 11, 397184,
                  11, 502239, 11, 490176
     LIST
     RUN
```

when asked for INPUT of the Chi-square value, enter
14.07.

Printout:

COMPARISON OF SEVERAL STANDARD DEVIATIONS
****

M= 11.5759

C= 1.0375

 THE TEST STATISTIC M/C= 11.1575

ENTER CHI-SQ. X2 FOR 7 DEG. FREEDOM

CHISQUARE VALUE= 14.07
 A-X2=-2.91251

 ACCEPT NULL HYPOTHESIS

Program MEAN1

(Text reference: §8.3 and §8.4, page 98)

Description: This program computes interval estimates
for a population mean from large and small samples.

Formulas used:

(i)   For sample size $N > 30$ the $(1-\alpha)$ level
confidence interval for the population
mean μ is

$$M - Z(\alpha/2)S/\sqrt{N} \leq \mu \leq M + Z(\alpha/2)S/\sqrt{N}$$

where M is the sample mean and S the sample standard
deviation (or population standard deviation, if
known).

For obtaining 90%, 95% or 99% confidence intervals
one should substitute 1.645, 1.96, or 2.576, for
$z(\alpha/2)$, respectively.

(ii) For sample size $N < 30$ the $(1-\alpha)$ level
confidence interval for μ is

$$M - t(\alpha/2)S/\sqrt{N} \leq \mu \leq M + t(\alpha/2)S/\sqrt{N}$$

where $t(\alpha/2)$ is that value of t with n-1 degrees of
freedom which is exceeded with probability $\alpha/2$, and
S is the sample standard deviation.

Data entry: Data lines are from 140 to 199 and data is
entered as

```
140  DATA  D, M, S, N
```

where

$$D = \begin{cases} 0 & \text{if } 1-\alpha = .95, \\ 1 & \text{if } 1-\alpha = .99, \\ 2 & \text{if } 1-\alpha = .90, \end{cases}$$

Program:

```
5 LPRINT"CONFIDENCE INTERVAL FOR MEAN"
6 LPRINT"*****************************"
7 LPRINT""
10 READ D,M,S,N
11 IF N<=30 THEN 100
15 LET S1=S/(SQR(N))
20 IF D=0 THEN 60
25 IF D=1 THEN 80
30 LET L1=M-1.645*S1
40 LET L2=M+1.645*S1
45 LPRINT"90% CONFIDENCE INTERVAL IS: "
50 LPRINT L1;"TO"L2 "INCLUDING END POINTS"
55 GOTO 10
58 LPRINT""
59 LPRINT""
60 LET L1=M-1.96*S1
65 LET L2=M+1.96*S2
69 LPRINT""
70 LPRINT"95% CONFIDENCE INTERVAL IS: "
75 GOTO 50
80 LET L1=M-2.576*S1
85 LET L2=M-2.576*S1
89 LPRINT""
90 LPRINT" 99%CONFIDENCE INTERVAL IS: "
95 GOTO 50
100 LPRINT"ENTER T=T(ALPHA/2) FOR";N-1;"DEG. OF FREEDOM"
105 INPUT T
110 LPRINT""
115 LPRINT"T VALUE="T
116 LPRINT""
120 LET L1=M-T*S/SQR(N)
125 LET L2=M+T*S/SQR(N)
130 LPRINT"REQUIRED CONFIDENCE INTERVAL IS:"
135 GOTO 50
250 END
```

Illustration 1. To find a 90% confidence interval for
the population mean when a random sample of size 40
has mean 25.5 and standard deviation 4.4, perform
the following:

```
LOAD "MEAN1"
140  DATA  2, 25.5, 4.4, 40
LIST
RUN
```

Printout:

CONFIDENCE INTERVAL FOR MEAN
****

90% CONFIDENCE INTERVAL IS:
 24.3556 TO 26.6444 INCLUDING END POINTS

Illustration 2. For Example 8.6 (page 100) first use
  program "DESC2" to obtain the sample mean and standard
  deviation. The steps to be performed are as follows:


```
     LOAD "DESC2"
     150  DATA  6, 2726, 2664, 2587, 2767, 2875, 2779
     LIST
     RUN
```


Printout:

COMPUTATION OF MEAN, VARIANCE, STD. DEVIATION
COEF. OF VARIATION AND STD. ERROR OF MEAN

NO OF OBSERVATIONS   6
MEAN   2733
STD. DEVIATION   99.5591
VARIANCE   9912
COEF. VARIATION   3.64285E-04
STD. ERROR OF MEAN   40.6448

Again perform the following:

```
     LOAD "MEAN1"
     140  DATA  2, 2733, 99.5591, 6
     LIST
     RUN
```

when asked for INPUT by the microcomputer enter
T = 2.571.

Printout:

```
CONFIDENCE INTERVAL FOR MEAN
****************************

ENTER T=T(ALPHA/2) FOR 5 DEG. OF FREEDOM

T VALUE= 2.571

REQUIRED CONFIDENCE INTERVAL IS:
 2628.5 TO 2837.5 INCLUDING END POINTS
```

Program MEAN2

(Text reference: §8.5, page 102)

Description: This program calculates the statistics
        needed to test the equality of two means when
        observations are paired.

Formula used: For sample size $N \leq 30$,

$$T = (M-F)/(S/\sqrt{N})$$

where M is the sample mean and S the sample standard
deviation of differences, and F the hypothesized
difference between the population means.

For sample size $N > 30$,

$$Z = (M-F)/(S/\sqrt{N})$$

Data entry: Data lines are from 71 to 149 and data is
  entered as

        75 DATA N, M, F, S

Program:

```
10 LPRINT" T-RATIO OR Z-VALUE FOR ONE SAMPLE "
15 LPRINT" ********************************** "
20 LPRINT""
25 READ N,M,F,S
30 IF N>30 GOTO 55
35 LET T=(M-F)/(S/SQR(N))
40 LPRINT"T-RATIO=";T;"WITH";N-1;"DEG. OF FREEDOM"
45 LPRINT""
50 GOTO 25
55 LET Z=(M-F)/(S/SQR(N))
60 LPRINT"OBSERVED Z=";Z
65 LPRINT""
70 GOTO 25
150 END
```

Illustration: Calculate the value of Z or T when

        (i)   N = 20, M = 6.03, F = 5.05, S = 3.74
        (ii) N = 150, M = 110.4, F = 112, S = 8 .

Perform the following:

```
LOAD "MEAN2"
75   DATA   20, 6.03, 5.05, 3.74
80   DATA   150, 110.4, 112, 8
LIST
RUN
```

Printout:

```
 T-RATIO OR Z-VALUE FOR ONE SAMPLE
 **********************************

T-RATIO = 1. 17184

OBSERVED Z=-2. 44949
```

Program MEAN3

(Text reference: §9.5(i), page 113)

Description: This program calculates the statistic
  needed to test the equality of two means when the
  population variances are unknown but assumed equal.

Formula used:

$$\text{t-ratio } T = \frac{M1 - M2}{S(\sqrt{1/N1 + 1/N2})}$$

where

$$S = \sqrt{\frac{(N1-1)S1^2 + (N2-1)S2^2}{N1 + N2 - 2}}$$

is the estimate of the common standard deviation,
N1, M1, S1 are the number of observations, mean
and standard deviation of sample 1, N2, M2, S2 are
the corresponding values for sample 2.

Degrees of freedom $V = N1 + N2 - 2$.

Data entry: Data lines are from 91 to 159 and data is
  entered as

        100   DATA   N1, M1, S1, N2, M2, S2

Program:

```
10 LPRINT"T-RATIO FOR TWO SAMPLES OR UNPAIRED T TEST"
15 LPRINT"********************************************"
20 LPRINT""
25 READ N1,M1,S1,N2,M2,S2
30 LET D=M1 - M2
35 LET L1 = (N1-1)*S1*S1
40 LET L2 = (N2-1)*S2*S2
45 LET S=SQR((L1+L2)/(N1+N2-2))
50 LET P=SQR((1/N1)+(1/N2))
55 LET T=D/(S*P)
60 LET R= INT(T*1000! + .5) /1000!
65 LET T1=ABS(R)
70 LPRINT"T-RATIO =";T1
75 LPRINT""
80 LPRINT"DEG. OF FREEDOM V = "; N1+N2-2
85 LPRINT""
90 GOTO 20
160 END
```

Example: The t-value for the data of Example 9.4
 (page 113) is obtained as follows:

Perform the following:

        LOAD "MEAN3"
        100   DATA 107, 173, 6.0, 87, 179, 7.0
        LIST
        RUN

Printout:

CALCULATION OF T RATIO FOR TWO SAMPLES OR UNPAIRED T-TEST
****

T-RATIO = 6.427

DEG. OF FREEDOM V = 192

Program MEAN4

(Text reference: §9.3(ii), pages 111 and 114)

Description: This program calculates the statistic
  needed to test the equality of two means when the
  population variances are either known or unknown
  and unequal.

Formulas used:

(i) If the population standard deviations are
     known and the sample sizes N1, N2 are not
     very small,

$$Z = \frac{(\bar{X}1 - \bar{X}2) - (M1 - M2)}{\sqrt{\frac{(S1)^2}{N1} + \frac{(S2)^2}{N2}}}$$

where $\bar{X}1$, $\bar{X}2$ are the sample means, M1, M2 the population
means, and S1 and S2 the population standard deviations.

(ii) If the standard deviations are unknown and
     can not be assumed equal,

$$U = \frac{(\bar{X}1 - \bar{X}2) - (M1 - M2)}{\sqrt{\frac{(S1)^2}{N1} + \frac{(S2)^2}{N2}}}$$

where S1 and S2 are sample standard deviations, is a
t-variable with degrees of freedom F1 given by

$$\frac{(S1^2/N1 + S2^2/N2)^2}{(S1^2/N1)^2/(N1-1) + (S2^2/N2)^2/(N2-1)}$$

Data entry: Data lines are from 86 to 199 and enter
  data as

    90 DATA D, N1, M1, S1, N2, M2, S2

where D is a dummy variable which is assigned the
value 0 if the population standard deviations are
known and a nonzero value if they are unknown and
unequal.

Program:

```
10 LPRINT"COMPUTING STATISTIC WHEN SAMPLE VARIANCE"
15 LPRINT"IS KNOWN OR UNKNOWN"
16 LPRINT"*******************************************"
20 READ D,N1,M1,S1,N2,M2,S2
25 LET A=S1*S1/N1
30 LET B=S2*S2/N2
35 LET U=(M1-M2)/SQR(A+B)
40 LPRINT""
45 LPRINT""
50 IF D=0 GOTO 80
55 LET F=(A+B)/((A*A/(N1-1))+(B*B/(N2-1)))
65 LPRINT"OBSERVED U=";U
70 LPRINT"NUMBER OF DEG. OF FREEDOM=";F
75 GOTO 20
80 LPRINT"OBSERVED Z=";U
85 GOTO 20
200 END
```

Illustration: We obtain the required statistics from
   Example 9.6 (page 115) by performing the following:

```
        LOAD "DESC2"
        150   DATA  14, 16.1, 16.8, 13.5, 13.0, 14.3,
                    11.6, 12.8
        155   DATA  17.5, 12.8, 8.9, 16.0, 16.8, 16.7,
                    15.2
        160   DATA  12, 14.6, 11.1, 7.0, 10.4, 15.8, 14.6
        165   DATA  9.4,9.8,5.1,5.5,6.4,7.1
        LIST
        RUN
```

Printout:

```
COMPUTATION OF MEAN, VARIANCE,STD. DEVIATION
COEF. OF VARIATION AND STD. ERROR OF MEAN
**************************************************

NO OF OBSERVATIONS        14
MEAN                      14.4286
STD. DEVIATION            2.45716
VARIANCE                  6.03762
COEF. VARIATION           1.70298E-03
STD. ERROR OF MEAN        .656703
```

```
NO OF OBSERVATIONS          12
MEAN                        9. 73333
STD. DEVIATION              3. 71125
VARIANCE                    13. 7734
COEF. VARIATION             3. 81293E-03
STD. ERROR OF MEAN          1. 07135
```

Now take the sample means and sample standard deviations as inputs in MEAN4 and perform:

```
LOAD "MEAN4"
90   DATA  1, 14, 14.4286, 2.45716, 12, 9.73333,
           3.71125
LIST
RUN
```

Printout:

```
COMPUTING STATISTIC WHEN SAMPLE VARIANCE
IS KNOWN OR UNKNOWN
***********************************************

OBSERVED U= 3. 73649
NUMBER OF DEG. OF FREEDOM= 11. 7777
```

Program MEAN5

(Text reference: §10.2, page 121)

Description: This program computes the F ratio for
   testing the equality of several population means
   on the basis of independent samples.

Formula used: Let

   K = number of samples

   $N(I)$ = number of items in the I-th sample
            $(I = 1,2,...,K)$

   $N = \Sigma_{I=1}^{K} N(I)$

Also let $X(1)$, $X(2)$, ..., $X(N)$ be the listing of all
items such that the first $N(1)$ of the X's constitute
the first sample, the next $N(2)$ items constitute the
second sample, etc. Let

$$V(I) = \Sigma_{j=1}^{N(I)} (Y(J))^2 - (\Sigma_{J=1}^{N(I)} Y(J))^2/N(I)$$

where $Y(1)$, $Y(2)$, ..., $Y(N(I))$ are items constituting
the ith sample.

Then the F-ratio $F = B/W$

where
$$B = \{\Sigma_{I=1}^{N}(X(I))^2 - (\Sigma_{I=1}^{N} X(I))^2/N - \Sigma_{I=1}^{N}V(I)\}/(K-1)$$

and

$$W = (\Sigma_{I=1}^{N} V(I))/(N-K).$$

Data entry: Data lines are from 250 to 299 and data is
   entered as

   250   DATA K, N(1), N(2), ..., N(K), X(1), X(2),...
               X(N)

Program:

```
2   LPRINT"THIS PROGRAM COMPUTES F-RATIO"
3   LPRINT"*********************************"
4   LPRINT""
5   DIM N(20),S(20),T(20),V(20),X(20)
10  READ K
15  LET N=0
20  LET S1=0
25  LET S2=0
30  FOR R=1 TO K
35  LET S(R)=0
40  LET T(R)=0
45  READ N(R)
50  LET N=N+N(R)
55  NEXT R
60  FOR J=1 TO K
65  FOR I=1 TO N(J)
70  READ X(I)
75  LET S(J)=S(J)+X(I)
80  LET T(J)=T(J)+X(I)*X(I)
90  LET S1=S1+X(I)
95  LET S2=S2+X(I)*X(I)
100 NEXT I
105 NEXT J
110 FOR I=1 TO K
120 LET V(I)=T(I)-(S(I)*S(I))/N(I)
125 LET S3=S3+V(I)
130 NEXT I
135 LET S4=S2-(S1*S1)/N
140 LET B1=S4-S3
145 LET B=B1/(K-1)
150 LET W=S3/(N-K)
155 LET F=B/W
170 LPRINT""
190 LPRINT" THE OBSERVED F RATIO IS ";F
195 LPRINT""
200 LPRINT""
205 LPRINT"DEGREES OF FREEDOM OF NUMERATOR="K-1
215 LPRINT""
220 LPRINT"DEGREES OF FREEDOM OF DENOMINATOR="N-K
225 GOTO 10
226 LPRINT""
300 END
```

Illustration: To calculate the F ratio for the data
  of Example 10.2 (page 122) perform the following:

```
        LOAD "MEAN5"
        250  DATA  4, 8, 15, 10, 12, 38, 5, 13, 18, 54, 66,
                   27
```

```
255   DATA   73, 62, 30, 78, 43, 45, 43, 40, 64, 43
260   DATA   32, 25, 61, 41, 65, 84, 75, 74, 58, 92
265   DATA   38, 30, 62, 62, 29, 82, 40, 82, 45
270   DATA   48, 59, 72, 78, 99, 36, 100, 87, 78
LIST
RUN
```

Printout:

```
THIS PROGRAM COMPUTES F-RATIO
*********************************

 THE OBSERVED F RATIO IS  4.02153


DEGREES OF FREEDOM OF NUMERATOR= 3

DEGREES OF FREEDOM OF DENOMINATOR= 41
```

Program PROB1

(Text reference: §4.4(i), page 58)

Description: This program computes the binomial probability of R successes in N independent trials.

Formula used: Probability $B = B(N;R;P) = \binom{N}{R}P^R(1-P)^{N-R}$
  where

  N = number of independent trials
  R = number of successes
  P = probability of success per trial
  $\binom{N}{R} = (N-R+1)(N-R+2)\ldots(N)/1.2\ldots.R$

Data entry: Data lines are from 121 to 199 and the data
  can be entered as

  130   DATA   N,R,P

Program:

```
10 LPRINT"#TRIALS", "#SUCC. ", "SUCC. PROB. ", "BINOM. PROB. "
11 LPRINT"******************************************************"
30 READ     N, R, P
35 LET S=(1-P)^N
40 IF R=0 THEN 90
45 LET H=1
50 FOR I=N-R+1 TO N
55 LET H=H*I
60 NEXT I
65 LET K=1
70 FOR L=1 TO R
75 LET K=K*L
80 NEXT L
85 LET S=(H/K)*(P^R)*((1-P)^(N-R))
90 LPRINT N, R, P, S
95 GOTO 30
200 END
```


Illustration: A suspension of Leishmania organisms was
  found to produce infection in 20% of the mice innocu-
  lated with it. If three mice are independently inno-
  culated, what are the probabilities that

  (i)   no mouse is infected;
  (ii) one mouse is infected;
  (iii) two mice are infected?

Perform the following:

```
LOAD "PROB1"
130   DATA  3,0,0.2
140   DATA  3, 1, 0.2
150   DATA  3, 2, 0.2
LIST
RUN
```

Printout:

#TRIALS	#SUCC.	SUCC. PROB.	BINOM. PROB.
3	0	.2	.512
3	1	.2	.384
3	2	.2	.096

Program PROB2

(Text reference: §4.4(i), page 63)

Description: This program computes the cumulative binomial probability of at most R successes.

Formula used:

$$\text{Probability} = \Sigma_{X=0}^{R} \ \binom{N}{X} \ P^X \ (1-P)^{N-X}$$

where

P = Probability of success per trial

$$\binom{N}{X} = (N-X+1)(N-X+2)\ldots(N)/1.2\ldots.X$$

Data entry: Data lines are from 121 to 299. Data should
be entered as

      230 DATA N,R,P

Program:

```
10 LPRINT"#TRIALS","#MAX. SUCC. ","SUCC. PROB. ","CUM. PROB. "
11 LPRINT"****************************************************"
30 READ     N,R,P
35 LET S=(1-P)^N
40 IF R=0 THEN 115
45 FOR I=1 TO R
50 LET K=1
65 LET H=1
70 FOR J=N-I+1 TO N
75 LET H= H*J
80 NEXT J
85 FOR L=1 TO I
90 LET K=K*L
95 NEXT L
100 LET B= (H/K)*(P^I)*((1-P)^(N-I))
105 LET S=S+B
110   NEXT I
115 LPRINT N,R,P,S
120 GOTO 30
200 END
```

Illustration: The probability that a flu vaccine will be
effective on any person is 0.7. If 4 people are selected
at random and injected with the vaccine,what is the probability that

      (a) at most two people will contract flu?
      (b) at most three people will contract flu?

Perform the following:

```
LOAD "PROB2"
230  DATA  4,2,.7
240  DATA  4,3,.7
LIST
RUN
```

Printout:

```
#TRIALS         #MAX. SUCC.    SUCC. PROB.    CUM. PROB.
***********************************************************
   4               2              .7             .3483
   4               3              .7             .7599
```

Program PROB3

(Text reference: §4.4(iii), page 64)

Description: This program enables one to use the normal
distribution table to approximate the probability of R
or more successes when the number of independent trials
is large.

Formulas used:

$$M = NP$$

$$S = \sqrt{(NP(1-P))}$$

$$Z1 = ((R-0.5)-M)/S$$

$$Z2 = ((R+0.5)-M)/S$$

where

N = number of independent trials
P = probability of success per trial.

If NP and N(1-P) $\geq$ 5 we approximate a binomial probability as follows:

(i) Probability of R successes in N trials = area
under the standard normal curve between Z1 and Z2.

(ii) Probability of at least R successes in N trials
= area under the standard normal curve to the right of Z1.

Data entry: Data lines are from 105 to 199 and data should
be entered as

110   DATA   D,N,P,R

where D is a dummy variable with D=0 when the
probability of exactly R successes is required and
D=1 when the probability of at least R successes is
required.

Program:

```
10 LPRINT"NORMAL APPROXIMATION TO BINOMIAL"
15 LPRINT"************************************"
20 LPRINT""
25 READ D,N,P,R
30 IF N*P < 5 THEN 95
35 IF N*(1-P) < 5 THEN 95
40 LET M=N*P
45 LET S=SQR(N*P*(1-P))
50 LET Z1=((R-.5)-M)/S
55 IF D=0 GOTO 75
60 LPRINT"PROBABILITY OF AT LEAST R SUCCESSES="
65 LPRINT"AREA OF NORMAL CURVE TO THE RIGHT OF Z="Z1
70 GOTO 20
71 LPRINT""
72 LPRINT""
75 LET Z2=((R+.5)-M)/S
80 LPRINT"PROBABILITY OF EXACTLY R SUCCESSES ="
81 LPRINT""
82 LPRINT""
85 LPRINT"AREA OF NORMAL CURVE BETWEEN";Z1;"AND";Z2
90 GOTO 20
92 LPRINT""
95 LPRINT"SAMPLE SIZE TOO SMALL FOR VALID APPROXIMATION"
100 GOTO 20
200 END
```

Illustration: To obtain the required probability for
  Example 4.8 (page 63) with the help of PROB3, observe
  that

$$P[10 \leq R \leq 15] = P[R \geq 10] - P[R \geq 16],$$

so we apply PROB3 to compute $P[R \geq 10]$ and $P[R \geq 16]$.

Perform the following:

```
LOAD "PROB3"
110  DATA  1,20,0.6,10
120  DATA  1,20,0.6,16
LIST
RUN
```

Printout:

```
NORMAL APPROXIMATION TO BINOMIAL
************************************

PROBABILITY OF AT LEAST R SUCCESSES=
AREA OF NORMAL CURVE TO THE RIGHT OF Z=-1.14109

PROBABILITY OF AT LEAST R SUCCESSES=
AREA OF NORMAL CURVE TO THE RIGHT OF Z= 1.59752
```

  In Table II, we can find the area under the standard
  normal curve between -1.14109 and 1.59752 in order to
  obtain the required probability.

Program PROB4

(Text reference: §4.4(iii), page 64)

Description: This program enables one to use the normal
   distribution table to approximate Poisson probabilities
   of R or more occurrences.

Formulas used:

$$S = \sqrt{M}$$
$$Z1 = ((R-0.5) - M)/S$$
$$Z2 = ((R+0.5) - M)/S$$

  where

        M = Mean of the Poisson variable.

We approximate Poisson probabilities as follows:

   (i)   Probability of R occurrences = area under the
          standard normal curve between Z1 and Z2.

   (ii)   Probability of at least R occurrences = Area
          under the standard normal curve to the right
          of Z1.

Data entry: Data lines are from 85 to 199 and data should
   be entered as

        110   DATA   D,M,R

where D is a dummy variable taking the value 0 in problems of type (i) above and the value 1 in problems of
type (ii).

Program:

```
10 LPRINT"NORMAL APPROXIMATION TO POISSON DISTRIBUTION"
15 LPRINT"************************************************"
20 LPRINT""
25 READ D,M,R
30 LET S=SQR(M)
35 LET Z1=((R-.5)-M)/S
40 IF D=0 THEN 60
45 LPRINT"PROBABILITY OF AT LEAST R SUCCESSES ="
50 LPRINT"AREA OF NORMAL CURVE TO THE RIGHT OF Z="Z1
55 GOTO 20
60 LET Z2=((R+.5)-M)/S
65 LPRINT"PROBABILITY OF EXACTLY R SUCCESSES ="
70 LPRINT"AREA OF NORMAL CURVE BETWEEN";Z1;"AND";Z2
80 GOTO 20
200 END
```

Illustration: (See page 63).   To approximate the probability that a Poisson variable with parameter M = 9 falls
   between 10 and 15 inclusive, proceed as follows:

```
     LOAD  "PROB4"
     110   DATA  1,9,10
     120   DATA  1,9,15
     LIST
     RUN
```

Printout:

NORMAL APPROXIMATION TO POISSON DISTRIBUTION
****

PROBABILITY OF AT LEAST R SUCCESSES =
AREA OF NORMAL CURVE TO THE RIGHT OF Z= .166667

PROBABILITY OF AT LEAST R SUCCESSES =
AREA OF NORMAL CURVE TO THE RIGHT OF Z= 1.83333

we can now look up the area under the standard normal
curve between .166667 & 1.83333 in Table II.

Program PROB5

(Text reference: §4.4, page 59)

Description: This program calculates the Poisson probability P of R occurrences

Formula used:

$$P = \exp(-M)\ R^M/R!$$

  where M is the average number of occurrences in a given
  unit of time or space.

Data entry: Data lines are from 101 to 199 and data should
  be entered as

      110   DATA   R,M

Program:


```
10 LPRINT"POISSON PROBABILITY"
15 LPRINT"*********************"
20 LPRINT""
25 LPRINT"#SUCCESS","MEAN VALUE","POISSON PROB."
30 LPRINT""
35 LPRINT""
40 READ R,M
45 IF R=0 GOTO 80
50 LET L=1
55 FOR I=1 TO R
60 LET L=L*I
65 NEXT I
70 LET P=(R^M)*EXP(-M)/L
75 GOTO 90
80 LET P=EXP(-M)
90 LPRINT R,M,P
95 LPRINT""
100 GOTO 40
200 END
```


Illustration: If the average rate of alarms at a fire
station between 5:00 to 9:00 PM is 1 per hour, what is
the probability of having

        (i)   no alarm between 5:00 PM and 6:00 PM?
        (ii) one fire alarm between 5:00 PM and 7:00 PM?

Perform the following:

```
LOAD "PROB5"
110   DATA  0,1
120   DATA  1,2
```

Printout:

```
POISSON PROBABILITY
*******************

#SUCCESS        MEAN VALUE      POISSON PROB.


0                 1               . 367879

1                 2               . 135335
```

Remark: In (ii), M was taken as 2, since the unit of
  time here is 2 hours.

Program PROB6

(Text reference:§4.4,page 59)

Description: This program computes the cumulative
  Poisson probability of at most R occurrences.

Formula used: Poisson probability of at most R
  occurrences =

$$\sum_{X=0}^{R} \exp(-M)M^{X}/X!$$

  where

    M = average number of occurrences per unit.

Data entry: Data lines are from 96 to 149 and data
  is entered as

    110 DATA R,M

Program:

```
5   LPRINT"CUMULATIVE POISSON PROBABILITY"
10  LPRINT"*******************************"
15  LPRINT""
20  LPRINT"#MAX. SUCC. ","AVG. SUCC. ","CUM. PROB. "
25  LPRINT""
30  LPRINT""
35  READ R,M
40  LET S=EXP(-M)
45  IF R=0 THEN 90
50  FOR I=1 TO R
55  LET K=1
60  FOR L=1 TO I
65  LET K=K*L
70  NEXT L
75  LET P=EXP(-M)*(M^I)/K
80  LET S=S+P
85  NEXT I
90  LPRINT R,M,S
95  GOTO 35
150 END
```

Illustration: For the fire alarm problem of Program
  PROB5, determine the probability of at most three
  alarms between 5 PM and 7 PM.

Perform the following:

```
LOAD"PROB6"
110 DATA 3,2
LIST
RUN
```

Printout:

```
CUMULATIVE POISSON PROBABILITY
*********************************

#MAX. SUCC.     AVG. SUCC.      CUM. PROB.


 3              2               857124
```

Program PROP1

(Text reference :§6.2,6.3,6.4(b), pages 77-79)

Description: This program computes the standard error
of a sample proportion and approximate confidence
intervals (at 90%,95%,99% levels) for a population
proportion.

Formulas used:

Proportion: $P = X/N$.
Standard error of proportion $P: \sqrt{X(N-X)/N^3}$.
Confidence interval with continuity correction:

$$P-Z\sqrt{P(1-P)/N} -1/(2N)\leq \pi \leq P+Z\sqrt{P(1-P)/N} +1/(2N)$$

where

X= number of elements belonging to the special
category,
N= sample size,
π= population proportion,
Z is a percentile of the standard normal variable
such that the area under the curve between $-Z$ and $+Z$ is
the confidence level.

Data entry: Data lines are from 121 to 209 and data is
entered as

130 DATA D,X,N

where D is a dummy variable with D=0 for a 95%
confidence level, D=1 for a 99% confidence level, D≠0,1
for a 90% confidence level.

Program:

```
5 LPRINT"APPROX. CONF. INTERVAL:CONTINUITY CORRECTION"
6 LPRINT"************************************************"
7 LPRINT""
10 READ D,X,N
15 LET P=X/N
20 LET S3=SQR(X*(N-X)/N^3)
25 LPRINT"STANDARD ERROR OF PROPORTION="S3
27 LPRINT""
30 LET S2=SQR(P*(1-P)/N)
35 IF D=0 THEN 55
40 IF D=1 THEN 65
45 LET L=1.645*S2
```

```
50 GOTO 70
55 LET L=1.96*S2
60 GOTO 70
65 LET L=2.576*S2
70 LET L1=P-L-1/(2*N)
75 LET L2=P+L+1/(2*N)
80 IF D=0 GOTO 105
85 IF D=1 GOTO 115
90 LPRINT"90% CONFIDENCE INTERVAL IS"
95 LPRINTL1;"TO";L2 "INCLUDING END POINTS"
97 LPRINT""
98 LPRINT""
100 GOTO 10
105 LPRINT"95% CONFIDENCE INTERVAL IS :"
110 GOTO 95
115 LPRINT"99% CONFIDENCE INTERVAL IS"
120 GOTO 95
200 END
```

Illustration: We calculate 90%,95% and 99% confidence
  intervals for the proportions given in Example 6.1
  (page 78). In this case X = 31,N = 60. We perform the
  following:

```
        LOAD"PROP1"
        130 DATA 2,31,60
        140 DATA 1,31,60
        150 DATA 0,31,60
        LIST
        RUN
```

Printout:

APPROX. CONF. INTERVAL:CONTINUITY CORRECTION
****

STANDARD ERROR OF PROPORTION= .0645138

90% CONFIDENCE INTERVAL IS
 .402208 TO .631125 INCLUDING END POINTS

STANDARD ERROR OF PROPORTION= .0645138

99% CONFIDENCE INTERVAL IS
 .342146 TO .691188 INCLUDING END POINTS

STANDARD ERROR OF PROPORTION= .0645138

95% CONFIDENCE INTERVAL IS :
 .381886 TO .651447 INCLUDING END POINTS

Program PROP2

(Text reference: §6.5, page 82)

Description: This program tests hypotheses about a
  proportion and prints out the values of the test
  statistic.

Formulas used:

(i)   If $(X-NP-.5)/\sqrt{NP(1-P)} > z(\alpha)$

we reject H_0: $p = P$ against H_R: $p > P$,

or H_0': $p \leq P$ against H_R: $p > P$.

(ii)   If $(X-NP+.5)/\sqrt{NP(1-P)} < -z(\alpha)$

we reject H_0: $p = P$ against H_L: $p < P$,

or H_0': $p \geq P$ against H_L: $p < P$.

(iii) If $(|X-NP| -.5)/\sqrt{NP(1-P)} > z(\alpha/2)$

we reject H_0: $p = P$ against H_T: $p \neq P$,
where

P = value of proportion under H_0,

X = number of elements in the sample belonging
    to the special category,

N = sample size,

α = level of significance.

Data entry: Data lines are from 131 to 199. Data is
  entered as

140   DATA D, P, X, N, Y

where D = 0,1,2 according as the test to be used is,
respectively, a right-tail, left-tail or a two-tail
test,

Y = $z(\alpha)$ if D = 0 or 1 and Y = $z(\alpha/2)$ if D = 2.

Remark: The following table gives values of Y for some commonly used levels of significance α.

Significance level α	Y value		
	Right tail	Left tail	Two tail
.1	1.28	1.28	1.64
.05	1.64	1.64	1.96
.025	1.96	1.96	2.24
.01	2.33	2.33	2.57
.005	2.57	2.57	2.81
.001	3.08	3.08	3.27

Program:

```
5   LPRINT"TEST OF HYPOTHESES OF A PROPORTION"
6   LPRINT"***********************************"
7   LPRINT""
10  READ D,P,X,N,Y
15  LET L=SQR(N*P*(1-P))
20  LET C=X-N*P
25  LET C1=(C-.5)/L
30  LET C2=(C+.5)/L
35  LET C3=(ABS(C)-.5)/L
40  IF D=0 THEN 90
45  IF D=1 THEN 110
50  LPRINT"COMPARE" C3 "WITH" Y
55  LPRINT""
60  LPRINT""
65  IF C3-Y >0 THEN 80
70  LPRINT"ACCEPT NULL HYPOTHESIS"
71  LPRINT""
72  LPRINT""
75  GOTO 10
80  LPRINT"REJECT NULL HYPOTHESIS"
81  LPRINT""
82  LPRINT""
85  GOTO 10
90  LPRINT"COMPARE" C1 "WITH" Y
92  LPRINT""
95  LPRINT""
100 IF C1-Y>0 THEN 80
105 GOTO 70
110 LPRINT"COMPARE" C2 "WITH" Y
115 LPRINT""
120 LPRINT""
125 IF C2+Y<0 THEN 80
130 GOTO 70
700 END
```

Illustration: To apply the above program to Example   6.3
  (page 82) perform the following:

```
LOAD "PROP2"
140   DATA  0, 0.1, 8, 50, 2.33
LIST
RUN
```

Printout:

TEST OF HYPOTHESES OF A PROPORTION
****

COMPARE 1.17851 WITH 2.33

ACCEPT NULL HYPOTHESIS

Program PROP3

(Text reference: §12.1, page 142)

Description: This program obtains 90%, 95%, 99% and
99.9% confidence intervals for the difference between
two proportions.

Formulas used:

Proportion P1 = X1/N1

Proportion P2 = X2/N2

where X1, X2 are the numbers of elements belonging to
the special category from samples of sizes N1 and N2,
respectively.

Confidence interval:

$$P1 - P2 \pm z(\alpha/2) \sqrt{\frac{X1(N1-X1)}{(N1)^3} + \frac{X2(N2-X2)}{(N2)^3}}$$

where $\alpha/2$ is the right tail area under the normal curve.

$z(\alpha/2)$ is 1.645, 1.96, 2.576 or 3.29

according as $1-\alpha$ is 90%, 95%, 99% or 99.9%.

Data entry: Data lines are from 180 to 299 and data is
entered as

190   DATA D, X1, N1, X2, N2

where D is a dummy variable which is assigned the
values 0,1,2 or 3 according as the confidence level
required is 95%, 99%, 99.9% or 90%.

Program:

```
5   LPRINT"CONFIDENCE INTERVAL FOR DIFFERENCE"
6   LPRINT"BETWEEN TWO PROPORTIONS"
10  LPRINT"****************************************"
11  LPRINT""
15  READ D
20  FOR I=1 TO 2
25  READ X(I),N(I)
30  LET P(I)=X(I)/N(I)
35  LET C(I)=X(I)*(N(I)-X(I))/(N(I)^3)
40  NEXT I
45  LET J=P(1)-P(2)
```

```
50 LET H=SQR(C(1)+C(2))
55 IF D=0 GOTO 80
60 IF D=1 GOTO 90
65 IF D=2 GOTO 100
66 LET K=1.645*H
70 GOTO 110
80 LET K=1.96*H
85 GOTO 110
90 LET K=2.576*H
95 GOTO 110
100 LET K=3.29*H
105 GOTO 110
110 LET L1 = J-K
120 LET L2=J+K
125 IF D=0 GOTO 147
130 IF D=1 GOTO 156
135 IF D=2 GOTO 166
136 LPRINT""
137 LPRINT""
140 LPRINT"90% CONFIDENCE INTERVAL IS :"
145 GOTO 175
147 LPRINT""
148 LPRINT""
150 LPRINT"95% CONFIDENCE INTERVAL IS : "
155 GOTO 175
156 LPRINT""
157 LPRINT""
160 LPRINT"99% CONFIDENCE INTERVAL IS: "
165 GOTO 175
166 LPRINT""
167 LPRINT""
170 LPRINT"99.9% CONFIDENCE INTERVAL IS : "
175 LPRINT L1;"TO";L2 "INCLUDING END POINTS"
176 GOTO 15
300 END
```

Illustration: We obtain the confidence intervals for
the data of Example 12.1 (page 144) as follows:

In that example $X1 = 16$, $N1 = 23$, $X2 = 9$, $N2 = 23$.

Perform the following:

```
LOAD "PROP3"
190   DATA  0, 16, 23, 9, 23
195   DATA  1, 16, 23, 9, 23
200   DATA  2, 16, 23, 9, 23
205   DATA  3, 16, 23, 9, 23
LIST
RUN
```

Printout:

CONFIDENCE INTERVAL FOR DIFFERENCE
BETWEEN TWO PROPORTIONS
****

95% CONFIDENCE INTERVAL IS :
 .0302202 TO .578476 INCLUDING END POINTS

99% CONFIDENCE INTERVAL IS:
-.0559341 TO .66463 INCLUDING END POINTS

99.9% CONFIDENCE INTERVAL IS :
-.155795 TO .764491 INCLUDING END POINTS

90% CONFIDENCE INTERVAL IS :
 .0742765 TO .534419 INCLUDING END POINTS

Program REGS1

(Text reference: §14.2, pages 163, 175)

Description: This program computes the linear regression
   equation and the correlation coefficient from an
   ungrouped sample

Formulas used:

      (i)   Regression line of Y on X:

          $Y = A + BX$

where

$$\text{Slope } B = \frac{N(\Sigma XY) - (\Sigma X)(\Sigma Y)}{N(\Sigma X^2) - (\Sigma X)^2}$$

Intercept $A = (\Sigma Y)/N - (B)(\Sigma X)/N$

      (ii)   Correlation coefficient:

$$R = B\sqrt{\frac{N(\Sigma X^2) - (\Sigma X)^2}{N(\Sigma Y^2) - (\Sigma Y)^2}}$$

Data entry: Data lines are from 160 to 299 and data is
   entered as

      160   DATA N, X(1), Y(1), ..., X(N), Y(N)

where N = number of observations.

Program:

```
10 LPRINT" COMPUTATION OF LINEAR REGRESSION EQUATION"
15 LPRINT" AND CORRELATION COEFFICIENT"
20 LPRINT"*****************************************************
25 LET X1=0
30 LET X2=0
35 LET Y1=0
40 LET Y2=0
45 LET Z1=0
50 READ N
55 FOR I=1 TO N
60 READ X,Y
```

```
65 LET X1=X1 + X
70 LET X2=X2 + X*X
75 LET Y1=Y1 + Y
80 LET Y2=Y2 + Y*Y
85 LET Z1=Z1 + X*Y
90 NEXT I
95 LET B=(N*Z1 - X1 * Y1)/(N*X2 - X1 * X1)
100 LET A= (Y1 / N) - B*(X1 / N)
105 LET R=B*SQR((N* X2 - X1 * X1 ) / (N * Y2 - Y1 * Y1 ))
110 IF B < 0 THEN 125
115 LPRINT" LIN REG EQUATION Y=";A;"+";B;"X"
120 GOTO 130
125 LPRINT" LIN REG EQUATION Y=";A;B;"X"
130 LPRINT""
135 LPRINT" CORR COEFFICIENT R=";R
140 LPRINT""
145 LPRINT""
150 GOTO 25
300 END
```

Illustration: Using the data of Example 14.7 (page 166),
   perform the following:

```
        LOAD "REGS1"
        200   DATA  5, 40, 120, 48, 115, 58, 140, 58,
                    125, 37, 110
        LIST
        RUN
```

Printout:


```
COMPUTATION OF LINEAR REGRESSION EQUATION
AND CORRELATION COEFFICIENT
*************************************************
 LIN REG EQUATION Y= 77. 157 + . 930353 X

CORR COEFFICIENT R= . 792734
```

Program REGS2

(Text reference: page 163)

Description: This program computes the best fitting
    linear, power, and exponential regression equations
    for a set of ungrouped data.

Formulas used:

(i)   Linear relationship: $Y = A + BX$

(ii)   Power relationship: $Y = A(X^B)$

(iii) Exponential relationship: $Y = A(e^{BX})$

The linear relationship is calculated as in REGS1.
The power and exponential relationships are reduced
to linear form by taking logarithms on each side of
the equation.

Data entry: Data lines are from 181 to 204. The data
    is entered as

185 DATA N, X(1), Y(1), ..., X(N), Y(N),

where N is the number of observations.

Program:

```
10 LPRINT" LEAST SQUARE CURVE FITTING"
15 REM LINEAR AND CURVILINEAR REGRESSION
20 LPRINT"**********************************"
25 LPRINT""
30 LPRINT""
35 LPRINT""
40 DIM K(100,2)
45 READ N
50 FOR I=1 TO N
55 READ K(I,1),K(I,2)
60 NEXT I
65 LPRINT" NO OF OBSERVATIONS N= ";N
70 LPRINT " DATA WERE ",  "   X",  " Y"
75 FOR I=1 TO N
80 LPRINT ,K(I,1),K(I,2)
85 NEXT I
90 DEF FN R(Z) = INT (Z * 1000! + .5)/ 1000!
91 LPRINT""
92 LPRINT""
93 GOSUB 280
94 LPRINT " LINEAR : Y=A+B*X "
95 LPRINT " WITH A= "; FN R(A);" AND B= "; FN R(B)
```

```
 96 LPRINT""
 97 LPRINT""
 98 FOR I= 1 TO N
 99 LET K(I,1)= LOG (K(I,1))
100 LET K(I,2) = LOG (K(I,2))
101 NEXT I
105 GOSUB 280
110 LPRINT "POWER : Y=A*(X^B) "
115 LPRINT "WITH A= "; FN R(EXP (A));"   AND B= "; FN R(B)
120 LPRINT""
125 LPRINT" CORR COEFFICIENT R= ";FN R(R)
130 LPRINT""
135 LPRINT""
140 FOR I=1 TO N
145 LET K(I,2)=LOG (K(I,2))
150 NEXT I
155 GOSUB 280
160 LPRINT "EXPONENTIAL : Y=A*EXP(B*X)"
165 LPRINT " WITH A= "; FN R(EXP (A)); " AND B= "; FN R(B)
170 LPRINT""
175 LPRINT "CORR COEFICIENT R= "; FN R(R)
180 LPRINT""
205 LPRINT""
210 LPRINT""
220 GOTO 45
225 STOP
280 LET S3=0
285 LET S4=0
290 LET S5=0
295 LET S6=0
300 LET S7=0
310 FOR I=1 TO N
315 LET S3=S3+K(I,1)
320 LET S4=S4+K(I,2)
325 LET S5=S5+K(I,1) * K(I,1)
330 LET S6=S6+K(I,2) * K(I,2)
335 LET S7=S7+K(I,1) * K(I,2)
340 NEXT I
345 LET B= (N * S7 -S3 * S4 )/ (N * S5 -S3 * S3 )
350 LET A= (S4 /N )-B * (S3 / N)
355 LET R= B* SQR ((N*S5 -S3 *S3 ) / (N * S6 -S4 *S4))
360 RETURN
```

Illustration: To find the best fitting linear, power
  and exponential regression functions for the following
  data:

(i)

X	6	10	12	15	17.8	24.0
Y	4	11.2	16	25	42.2	64

(ii)

X	1.6	1.8	2.0	2.2	2.4	2.6
Y	2.47	2.07	1.77	1.53	1.35	1.19

(iii)

X	3	4	5	6	7	8
Y	9.96	14.85	22.2	33	49.4	73.6

Perform the following:

```
LOAD "REGS2"
185  DATA  6, 6, 4, 10, 11.2, 12, 16, 15, 25, 17,
           8, 42.2, 24.0, 64
195  DATA  6, 1.6, 2.47, 1.8, 2.07, 2.0, 1.77, 2.2,
           1.53, 2.4, 1.35, 2.6, 1.19
200  DATA  6, 3, 9.96, 4, 14.85, 5, 22.2, 6, 33, 7,
           49.4, 8, 73.6
LIST
RUN
```

Printout:

```
LEAST SQUARE CURVE FITTING
***********************************


NO OF OBSERVATIONS N=  6


DATA WERE       X               Y
                6               4
                10              11. 2
                12              16
                15              25
                17. 8           42. 2
                24              64


 LINEAR : Y=A+B*X
 WITH A= -22. 204   AND B=  3. 486


POWER : Y=A*(X^B)
WITH A=  . 101    AND B=  2. 048

 CORR COEFFICIENT R=  . 998


EXPONENTIAL · Y=A*EXP(B*X)
 WITH A=  . 358   AND B=  . 802

CORR COEFICIENT R=  . 984
```

```
 NO OF OBSERVATIONS N=  6
 DATA WERE       X             Y
                 1. 6          2. 47
                 1. 8          2. 07
                 2            1. 77
                 2. 2          1. 53
                 2. 4          1. 35
                 2. 6          1. 19


 LINEAR :  Y=A+B*X
 WITH A=   4. 37   AND B= -1. 257


POWER :  Y=A*(X^B)
WITH A=  5    AND B= -1. 5

 CORR COEFFICIENT R= -1


EXPONENTIAL :  Y=A*EXP(B*X)
 WITH A=   4. 807   AND B= -3. 251

CORR COEFICIENT R= -. 971


 NO OF OBSERVATIONS N=  6

 DATA WERE       X             Y
                 3            9. 96
                 4            14. 85
                 5            22. 2
                 6            33
                 7            49. 4
                 8            73. 6


 LINEAR :  Y=A+B*X
 WITH A= -34. 153   AND B=  12. 361


POWER :  Y=A*(X^B)
WITH A=  . 95   AND B=  2. 028

 CORR COEFFICIENT R=   . 99


EXPONENTIAL :  Y=A*EXP(B*X)
 WITH A=  1. 122   AND B=  . 639

CORR COEFICIENT R=   . 999
```

Program REGS3

(Text reference: §14.2, §14.3, page 173)

Description: In addition to the regression equation and
  correlation coefficient, this program computes the
  standard deviation about the regression line, standard
  errors of the slope and intercept, 95% confidence limits
  for the population regression line and the t-ratio for
  the correlation coefficient R.

Formulas used:

(i)   Mean of X: $M1 = \Sigma X/N$, Mean of Y: $M2 = \Sigma Y/N$.

(ii)   Regression line: $Y = A + BX$, with A and B
       as in Program REGS1.

(iii) Correlation coefficient: R as in Program
       REGS1.

(iv)   For testing whether R is significantly
       different from 0,

$$T1 = R \sqrt{(N-2)/(1-R^2)}$$

       has a t-distribution with N-2 degrees of
       freedom.

(v)   Standard deviation D of the data points
       about the regression line:

$$D = \sqrt{(1-R^2)(\Sigma Y^2 - (\Sigma Y)^2/N)/(N-2)}.$$

(vi)   Standard error of the intercept A:

$$E1 = D.\sqrt{(1/N)+(\Sigma X/N)^2/(\Sigma X^2-(\Sigma X)^2/N)}$$

(vii) Standard error of the slope B:

$$E2 = D/\sqrt{\{\Sigma X^2-(\Sigma X)^2/N\}}.$$

Confidence limits corresponding to any given value
of X:

$$\text{Upper } Y = M2+B(X-M1)+t(\alpha/2).D\sqrt{\frac{1}{N} + \frac{(M1-X)^2}{\Sigma X^2-(\Sigma X)^2/N}}$$

$$\text{Lower } Y = M2-B(X-M1)-t(\alpha/2).D\sqrt{\frac{1}{N} + \frac{(M1-X)^2}{\Sigma X^2-(\Sigma X)^2/N}}$$

where $t(\alpha/2)$ is obtained from the table for t
distributions with N-2 degrees of freedom. When
α = .05 we get 95% confidence limits.

Data entry: Data lines are from 350 to 449 and data
is entered as

        350 DATA N, X(1), Y(1), ..., X(N), Y(N)

where N is the number of observations.

Program:

```
10 LPRINT"REGRESSION, CORRELATION AND ASSOC.  STATISTICS"
15 LPRINT"**************************************************"
20 LPRINT""
25 LPRINT""
30 LPRINT""
35 DIM P(100),Q(100)
40 READ N
45 LPRINT" ENTER T (AT P=0.05) FOR N-2 DEG OF FREEDOM "
50 INPUT T
55 LPRINT"T=";T
60 FOR I=1 TO N
65 READ P(I),Q(I)
70 NEXT I
75 LET X1 = 0
80 LET X2 = 0
85 LET Y1 = 0
90 LET Y2 = 0
95 LET Z=0
100 FOR I= 1 TO N
105 LET X1=X1 +P(I)
110 LET Y1=Y1 +Q(I)
115 LET X2= X2 + P(I)*P(I)
120 LET Y2= Y2 + Q(I)*Q(I)
125 LET Z=Z+P(I) * Q(I)
130 NEXT I
135 LPRINT""
140 LET M1 = X1 / N
145 LET M2 = Y1 / N
150 LET B= ( N*Z -X1 * Y1) / (N*X2 -X1 * X1)
155 LET A=M2 -B * M1
160 LET R=B* SQR ((N * X2 -X1 * X1)/(N*Y2 - Y1 * Y1))
165 DEF FN R(V) = INT ( V * 1000! + .5 ) /1000!
170 LPRINT" NO OF OBSERVATIONS  ";N
```

```
175 LPRINT" MEAN OF X "; FN R(M1)" MEAN OF Y   "; FN R(M2)
180 LPRINT""
185 LPRINT" REGRESSION EQUATION Y=A+B*X"
190 LPRINT " WITH A  "; FN R(A)" AND B  "; FN R(B)
195 LPRINT""
200 LET F= Y2 - ((Y1 * Y1)/N)
205 LET G= X2 - ((X1 * X1)/N)
210 LET H= 1- R*R
215 LET D= SQR ((H/(N-2))*F)
220 LET E1=D*SQR(1/N + (M1*M1)/G)
225 LET E2= D/SQR (G)
230 LET T1= R * SQR ((N-2) / H)
235 LPRINT""
240 LPRINT"STD DEV ABOUT REG LINE   "; FN R(D)
245 LPRINT" STD ERROR OF A  "; FN R(E1)
250 LPRINT" STD ERROR OF B  "; FN R(E2)
255 LPRINT""
260 LPRINT" CORR COEFFICIENT R   "; FN R(R)
265 LPRINT" T VALUE FOR R "; FN R(T1)
270 LPRINT""
280 LPRINT "X", "Y"; "          ";"95%CONFIDENCE LIMITS
281 LPRINT "*****************************************"
285 DEF FN R(C) = INT(C * 10! + .5) /10!
290 FOR I=1 TO N
295 LET W= (T*D)*SQR ((1/N + ((M1-P(I)) ^ 2 /G)/G))
300 LET U=M2 + B* (P(I) - M1) + W
305 LET L=M2 + B * (P(I) - M1) -W
310 LPRINT FNR(P(I)),FNR(Q(I));"    "FNR(U);"    "FNR(L)
315 NEXT I
320 GOTO 40
450 END
```

Illustration: To obtain the regression line, standard
   deviation about the regression line and 95% confidence
   limits from the data

        X = 2, 2, 3, 3, 3, 4, 4, 4, 5

        Y = 2, 3, 2, 3, 4, 3, 4, 5, 5

Perform the following:

        LOAD "REGS3"
        350 DATA 9, 2, 2, 2, 3, 3, 2, 3, 3, 3, 4, 4,
                   3, 4, 4, 4, 5, 5, 5
        LIST
        RUN

   The following printout is obtained after we input
   T(.05) = 2.365

Printout:

REGRESSION, CORRELATION AND ASSOC. STATISTICS

****

  ENTER T (AT P=0.05) FOR N-2 DEG OF FREEDOM
T= 2.365

  NO OF OBSERVATIONS   9
  MEAN OF X   3.333   MEAN OF Y   3.444

  REGRESSION EQUATION Y=A+B*X
  WITH A   .667   AND B   .833

STD DEV ABOUT REG LINE   .816
  STD ERROR OF A   1
  STD ERROR OF B   .289

  CORR COEFFICIENT R   .737
  T VALUE FOR R   2.887

X   Y   95%CONFIDENCE LIMITS
****
  2   2   3.1   1.6
  2   3   3.1   1.6
  3   2   3.8   2.5
  3   3   3.8   2.5
  3   4   3.8   2.5
  4   3   4.7   3.3
  4   4   4.7   3.3
  4   5   4.7   3.3
  5   5   5.6   4.1

Program REGS4

(Text reference: §14.7, page 179)

Description: This program computes Spearman's rank
  correlation coefficient R_s.

Formula used:

$$R = 1 - 6 \sum_{I=1}^{N} D^2(I)/N(N-1)(N+1)$$

where

$D(I) = X(I) - Y(I)$

$X(I)$, $Y(I)$ $(I = 1,2,...,N)$ are the observations,

N = number of observations.

Data entry: Data lines are from 130 to 199 and the data
  can be entered as

140   DATA N, X(1), Y(1), ..., X(N), Y(N)

Program:

```
10 DIM X(50),Y(50),D(50)
20 LPRINT"SPEARMANS RANK CORRELATION COEFFICIENT"
25 LPRINT"****************************************"
28 LPRINT""
30 READ N
40 LET D2=0
50 FOR I=1 TO N
60 READ X(I),Y(I)
70 LET D(I)=X(I)-Y(I)
80 LET D2=D2+D(I)*D(I)
90 NEXT I
100 LET R=1-6*(D2)/(N*(N-1)*(N+1))
107 LPRINT""
110 LPRINT"SPEARMANS RANK CORR. COEFF. = ";R
120 GOTO 30
200 END
```

Illustration: Using the data of Example 14.11 (page 178)
  perform the following:

```
LOAD "REGS4"
130    DATA   39, 16, 12, 14, 20, 17.5, 18, 31.5, 19,
               25, 23
135    DATA   31.5, 25, 20, 14, 10, 11, 19, 28, 26, 33,
               22, 22
```

```
140   DATA   34, 35, 35, 38, 33, 32, 11, 3, 37, 15.5,
             15, 17
145   DATA   39, 39, 28, 31, 27, 29, 23, 30, 21, 26,
             30, 27
150   DATA   13, 24, 24, 21, 38, 36, 29, 24, 36, 37,
             17.5, 15.5
155   DATA   8, 9, 5, 7, 9, 2, 7, 10, 2, 4, 1, 6, 6,
             8, 4, 1, 3, 5, 12, 13
LIST
RUN
```

Printout:

SPEARMANS RANK CORRELATION COEFFICIENT
****

SPEARMANS RANK CORR. COEFF. =   .865081

Program SIGNT

(Text reference: §16.2, page 201)

Description: This program carries out the Sign Test
  for a set of paired numerical observations.

Formulas used:

   (i)   If $(2R-N-1)/\sqrt{N} > Z(\alpha)$ reject H_0 against
          right-sided alternatives.

   (ii)   If $(2R-N+1)/\sqrt{N} < -Z(\alpha)$ reject H_0 against
          left-sided alternatives.

   (iii) If $(|2R-N| - 1)/\sqrt{N} > Z(\alpha/2)$ reject H_0
          against two-sided alternatives, where

   N = number of paired samples with unequal $X(I)$
       and $Y(I)$,

   R = number of positive $X(I) - Y(I)$'s
       $(I = 1,2,\ldots,N)$,

   α = level of significance.

  The value of z for the right, left or two-tail tests
is obtained from the table given in PROP2.

Data entry: Data lines are from 165 to 245 and enter
  data as

      165 DATA D, S, N, X(1), Y(1), ..., X(N), Y(N)

  where D is a dummy variable which is assigned a value
0, 1 or 2 according as the alternatives are right,
left, or two-sided,

      S = significance level α,

      N = Number of unequal values of X and Y,

  $X(I)$, $Y(I)$ are the pairwise different values of X
and Y for $I = 1,2,\ldots,N$.

Program:

```
10 LPRINT"SIGN TEST: HYPOTHESIS TESTING"
11 LPRINT"********************************"
15 DIM X(20),Y(20),D(20)
20 READ D,S,N
25 LET R=0
30 FOR I=1 TO N
35 READ X(I),Y(I)
36 LET D(I)=X(I)-Y(I)
42 IF D(I)<=0 THEN 50
45 R=R+1
50 NEXT I
55 LET C=2*R-N
60 LET E=SQR(N)
65 LET C1=(C-.5)/E
70 LET C2=(C+.5)/E
75 LET C3=(ABS(C)-.5)/E
80 IF D=0 THEN 125
85 IF D=1 THEN 145
90 LPRINT"COMPARE";C3;"WITH Z(ALPHA/2)="S
95 LPRINT""
100 IF C3-S>0 THEN 115
105 LPRINT"ACCEPT THE NULL HYPOTHESIS"
110 GOTO 20
115 LPRINT"REJECT THE NULL HYPOTHESIS"
120 GOTO 20
125 LPRINT"COMPARE";C1;"WITH Z(ALPHA)="S
130 LPRINT""
135 IF C1-Y>0 THEN 115
140 GOTO 105
145 LPRINT"COMPARE";C2;"WITH Z(ALPHA)="S
150 LPRINT""
155 IF C2+Y>0 THEN 115
160 GOTO 105
250 END
```

Illustration: To apply the program SIGNT to the data
   of Example 16.1 (page 201) we first observe that
   the test required is a right tail test. Let the
   level of significance be α = .05 then for a one tail
   test $z_{.05}$ = 1.64. Now perform the following

```
LOAD "SIGNT'
165   DATA  0, 1.64, 10, 16.5, 13.8, 10.0, 9.9,
            16.4, 16.7
170   DATA  22.0, 22.5, 34.5, 24.5, 9.0, 9.3, 12.6,
            12.8
```

```
175   DATA   12.7, 11.5, 12.0, 15.5, 9.9, 11.0, 59,
             59
LIST
RUN
```

Printout:

```
SIGN TEST: HYPOTHESIS TESTING
********************************
COMPARE-.790569 WITH Z(ALPHA)= 1.64

ACCEPT THE NULL HYPOTHESIS
```

APPENDIX
Statistical Tables and Frequently Used Symbols

Table I

Table of Random Digits

86197	86833	93718	97418	33814	25950	87053	70680	92122	12833
70333	18483	83972	80902	37839	19059	42974	49571	92994	23638
71403	59913	08129	51255	70615	59040	13703	89626	33252	78067
36094	52078	64338	77373	94711	19731	46920	54756	47643	27810
16514	16934	06606	25170	79782	22088	98948	54198	84220	66005
08845	48800	25666	38178	77394	94552	19439	59351	54890	26978
36091	02146	99117	21494	80062	52857	43467	64694	31234	39234
31383	25599	12441	64661	12182	60977	24372	72972	23732	38130
81971	56906	87013	02056	50191	78937	29932	57544	33898	24585
85422	46270	13765	84643	42695	57102	38206	82957	82437	35891
02889	69618	72475	17768	62088	49737	44873	79110	03320	21175
01450	36512	32080	65737	30571	69319	85084	27925	97538	91189
97521	73530	00748	37300	89128	36857	82210	16933	48671	90769
10918	48275	89687	08341	20277	74071	33859	98779	36198	93714
94220	14850	67303	98337	18838	17946	16394	28299	23630	29293
24066	59885	93188	99399	16009	51281	52542	77511	18106	62483
03443	40382	33485	46907	80006	19092	10590	40823	26566	34580
17699	88138	22670	30391	25437	09440	56138	13114	09068	85328
33093	33878	59113	82593	39219	30046	89549	21019	33320	25631
42538	25810	42082	96351	80980	78321	71010	12120	20639	06725
16704	00158	39842	09802	47463	93317	90860	23345	00311	52334
07484	93811	77385	25828	40352	25154	03929	24525	46099	24766
23246	40749	40684	36526	82189	26839	29527	50440	29002	14548
33540	62795	47638	74186	33287	37801	74769	92992	56963	05211
08096	51916	15997	56080	16801	43494	64929	84526	67824	21202
72151	94848	12014	78928	26135	45610	35731	64549	04160	23462
88378	77184	91864	93873	83426	23947	99199	39407	23969	76458
09747	75188	51979	60516	86766	27558	72844	55046	79955	30671
58099	28292	70023	69064	58905	55103	27776	22064	32460	71176
21103	55968	62231	27750	26763	89844	48482	70989	93564	14791
94074	97199	59829	92784	36801	06952	35317	92756	96235	68294
79596	77574	99949	19593	97951	36966	90680	96969	00602	98791
38511	66740	13344	84268	50168	34294	07004	00708	50549	43333
15348	35606	79741	50767	48656	99076	09287	35785	85289	78500
74941	66846	63690	38296	19612	42571	52489	32149	70200	62189
63285	93535	53599	54569	05687	10903	54964	84815	05247	62840
02207	87384	36296	13588	88294	94437	81705	53809	66033	99650
86004	51644	99532	12922	67736	65091	58150	09908	95956	03317
38065	02458	70597	76457	85314	12657	70279	99925	59352	73413
08015	48668	65479	43442	30729	52246	57930	31116	03122	31170
59049	01077	81222	96191	62177	27472	33128	08208	00605	08802
71707	10023	13968	31411	10205	19199	04550	81521	46608	37389
00221	94118	66572	13460	73609	01421	54137	51235	40768	66121
38074	06127	80349	79806	99898	98412	11371	16985	47364	05026
54201	80543	20229	83026	18573	50600	14382	39560	60622	91069

Table II

Probabilities of the Standard Normal Variable

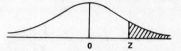

This table gives, for each specified z, the probability that the standard normal variable exceeds z.

Z	.00	.01	.02	.03	.04	.05	.06	.07	.08	.09
0.0	.5000	.4960	.4920	.4880	.4840	.4801	.4761	.4721	.4681	.4641
0.1	.4602	.4562	.4522	.4483	.4443	.4404	.4364	.4325	.4286	.4246
0.2	.4207	.4168	.4129	.4090	.4052	.4013	.3974	.3936	.3897	.3859
0.3	.3821	.3783	.3745	.3707	.3669	.3632	.3594	.3557	.3520	.3483
0.4	.3446	.3409	.3372	.3336	.3300	.3264	.3228	.3192	.3156	.3121
0.5	.3085	.3050	.3015	.2981	.2946	.2912	.2877	.2843	.2810	.2776
0.6	.2742	.2709	.2676	.2644	.2611	.2578	.2546	.2514	.2482	.2451
0.7	.2420	.2388	.2358	.2327	.2296	.2266	.2236	.2206	.2177	.2148
0.8	.2119	.2090	.2061	.2033	.2004	.1977	.1949	.1922	.1894	.1867
0.9	.1841	.1814	.1788	.1762	.1736	.1711	.1685	.1660	.1635	.1611
1.0	.1587	.1562	.1539	.1515	.1492	.1469	.1446	.1423	.1401	.1379
1.1	.1357	.1335	.1314	.1292	.1271	.1251	.1230	.1210	.1190	.1170
1.2	.1151	.1131	.1112	.1094	.1075	.1056	.1038	.1020	.1003	.0985
1.3	.0968	.0951	.0934	.0918	.0901	.0885	.0869	.0853	.0838	.0823
1.4	.0808	.0793	.0778	.0764	.0749	.0735	.0721	.0708	.0694	.0681
1.5	.0668	.0655	.0642	.0630	.0618	.0606	.0594	.0582	.0571	.0559
1.6	.0548	.0537	.0526	.0516	.0505	.0495	.0485	.0475	.0465	.0455
1.7	.0446	.0436	.0427	.0418	.0409	.0401	.0392	.0384	.0375	.0367
1.8	.0359	.0351	.0344	.0336	.0329	.0322	.0314	.0307	.0301	.0294
1.9	.0287	.0281	.0274	.0268	.0262	.0256	.0250	.0244	.0239	.0233
2.0	.0228	.0222	.0217	.0212	.0207	.0202	.0197	.0192	.0188	.0183
2.1	.0179	.0174	.0170	.0166	.0162	.0158	.0154	.0150	.0146	.0143
2.2	.0139	.0136	.0132	.0129	.0125	.0122	.0119	.0116	.0113	.0110
2.3	.0107	.0104	.0102	.0099	.0096	.0094	.0091	.0089	.0087	.0084
2.4	.0082	.0080	.0078	.0075	.0073	.0071	.0069	.0068	.0066	.0064
2.5	.0062	.0060	.0059	.0057	.0055	.0054	.0052	.0051	.0049	.0048
2.6	.0047	.0045	.0044	.0043	.0041	.0040	.0039	.0038	.0037	.0036
2.7	.0035	.0034	.0033	.0032	.0031	.0030	.0029	.0028	.0027	.0026
2.8	.0026	.0025	.0024	.0023	.0023	.0022	.0021	.0021	.0020	.0019
2.9	.0019	.0018	.0018	.0017	.0016	.0016	.0015	.0015	.0014	.0014
3.0	.0013	.0013	.0013	.0012	.0012	.0011	.0011	.0011	.0010	.0010

Table II is taken from Table II1 of Fisher and Yates' *Statistical Tables for Biological, Agricultural and Medical Research,* published by Longman Group Ltd., London, (previously published by Oliver & Boyd Ltd., Edinburgh) and by permission of the authors and publishers.

Table III
Percentile Points of Chi-Square Variables

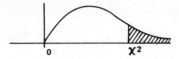

Corresponding to each specified upper tail probability P, this table gives that value of the Chi-square variable with r degrees of freedom which is exceeded with probability P

P r	0.990	0.975	0.950	0.900	0.250	0.100	0.050	0.025	0.010
1	0.0^3157	0.0^3982	0.0^2393	0.0158	1.323	2.706	3.841	5.024	6.635
2	0.020	0.051	0.103	0.211	2.773	4.605	5.991	7.378	9.210
3	0.115	0.216	0.352	0.584	4.108	6.251	7.815	9.348	11.345
4	0.297	0.484	0.711	1.064	5.385	7.779	9.488	11.143	13.277
5	0.554	0.831	1.145	1.610	6.626	9.236	11.070	12.832	15.086
6	0.872	1.237	1.635	2.204	7.841	10.645	12.592	14.449	16.812
7	1.239	1.690	2.167	2.833	9.037	12.017	14.067	16.013	18.475
8	1.646	2.180	2.733	3.490	10.219	13.362	15.507	17.535	20.090
9	2.088	2.700	3.325	4.168	11.389	14.684	16.919	19.023	21.666
10	2.558	3.247	3.940	4.865	12.549	15.987	18.307	20.483	23.209
11	3.053	3.816	4.575	5.578	13.701	17.275	19.675	21.920	24.725
12	3.571	4.404	5.226	6.304	14.845	18.549	21.026	23.337	26.217
13	4.107	5.009	5.892	7.042	15.984	19.812	22.362	24.736	27.688
14	4.660	5.629	6.571	7.790	17.117	21.064	23.685	26.119	29.141
15	5.229	6.262	7.261	8.547	18.245	22.307	24.996	27.488	30.578
16	5.812	6.908	7.962	9.312	19.369	23.542	26.296	28.845	32.000
17	6.408	7.564	8.672	10.085	20.489	24.769	27.587	30.191	33.409
18	7.015	8.231	9.390	10.865	21.605	25.989	28.869	31.526	34.805
19	7.633	8.907	10.117	11.651	22.718	27.204	30.144	32.852	36.191
20	8.260	9.591	10.851	12.443	23.828	28.412	31.410	34.170	37.566
21	8.897	10.283	11.591	13.240	24.935	29.615	32.670	35.479	38.932
22	9.542	10.982	12.338	14.042	26.039	30.813	33.924	36.781	40.289
23	10.196	11.688	13.090	14.848	27.141	32.007	35.172	38.076	41.638
24	10.856	12.401	13.848	15.659	28.241	33.196	36.415	39.364	42.980
25	11.52	13.12	14.61	16.47	29.34	34.38	37.65	40.65	44.31
26	12.20	13.84	15.38	17.29	30.43	35.56	38.89	41.92	45.64
27	12.88	14.57	16.15	18.11	31.53	36.74	40.11	43.19	46.96
28	13.56	15.31	16.93	18.94	32.62	37.92	41.34	44.46	48.28
29	14.26	16.05	17.71	19.77	33.71	39.09	42.56	45.72	49.59
30	14.95	16.79	18.49	20.60	34.80	40.26	43.77	46.98	50.89
40	22.16	24.43	26.51	29.05	45.62	51.80	55.76	59.34	63.69
50	29.71	32.36	34.76	37.69	56.33	63.17	67.50	71.42	76.15
60	37.48	40.48	43.19	46.46	66.98	74.40	79.08	83.30	88.38
70	45.44	48.76	51.74	55.33	77.58	85.53	90.53	95.02	100.42
80	53.54	57.15	60.39	64.28	88.13	96.58	101.88	106.63	112.33
90	61.75	65.65	69.13	73.29	98.65	107.56	113.14	118.14	124.12
100	70.06	74.22	77.93	82.36	109.14	118.50	124.34	129.56	135.81

Table IV
Percentage Points of Student's t

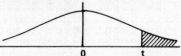

Corresponding to each specified upper tail probability P, this table gives that value of the t variable with r degrees of freedom which is exceeded with probability P.

P r	·25	·10	·05	·025	·01	·005
1	1·000	3·078	6·314	12·706	31·821	63·657
2	0·816	1·886	2·920	4·303	6·965	9·925
3	·765	1·638	2·353	3·182	4·541	5·841
4	·741	1·533	2·132	2·776	3·747	4·604
5	0·727	1·476	2·015	2·571	3·365	4·032
6	·718	1·440	1·943	2·447	3·143	3·707
7	·711	1·415	1·895	2·365	2·998	3·499
8	·706	1·397	1·860	2·306	2·896	3·355
9	·703	1·383	1·833	2·262	2·821	3·250
10	0·700	1·372	1·812	2·228	2·764	3·169
11	·697	1·363	1·796	2·201	2·718	3·106
12	·695	1·356	1·782	2·179	2·681	3·055
13	·694	1·350	1·771	2·160	2·650	3·012
14	·692	1·345	1·761	2·145	2·624	2·977
15	0·691	1·341	1·753	2·131	2·602	2·947
16	·890	1·337	1·746	2·120	2·583	2·921
17	·689	1·333	1·740	2·110	2·567	2·898
18	·688	1·330	1·734	2·101	2·552	2·878
19	·688	1·328	1·729	2·093	2·539	2·861
20	0·687	1·325	1·725	2·086	2·528	2·845
21	·686	1·323	1·721	2·080	2·518	2·831
22	·686	1·321	1·717	2·074	2·508	2·819
23	·685	1·319	1·714	2·069	2·500	2·807
24	·685	1·318	1·711	2·064	2·492	2·797
25	0·684	1·316	1·708	2·060	2·485	2·787
26	·684	1·315	1·706	2·056	2·479	2·779
27	·684	1·314	1·703	2·052	2·473	2·771
28	·683	1·313	1·701	2·048	2·467	2·763
29	·683	1·311	1·699	2·045	2·462	2·756
30	0·683	1·310	1·697	2·042	2·457	2·750
40	·681	1·303	1·684	2·021	2·423	2·704
60	·679	1·296	1·671	2·000	2·390	2·660
120	·677	1·289	1·658	1·980	2·358	2·617
∞	·674	1·282	1·645	1·960	2·326	2·576

Table Va

Upper 5% Points of the F distribution

r \ s	1	2	3	4	5	6	7	8	9	10	12	15	20	24	30	40	60	120	∞
1	161·4	199·5	215·7	224·6	230·2	234·0	236·8	238·9	240·5	241·9	243·9	245·9	248·0	249·1	250·1	251·1	252·2	253·3	254·3
2	18·51	19·00	19·16	19·25	19·30	19·33	19·35	19·37	19·38	19·40	19·41	19·43	19·45	19·45	19·46	19·47	19·48	19·49	19·50
3	10·13	9·55	9·28	9·12	9·01	8·94	8·89	8·85	8·81	8·79	8·74	8·70	8·66	8·64	8·62	8·59	8·57	8·55	8·53
4	7·71	6·94	6·59	6·39	6·26	6·16	6·09	6·04	6·00	5·96	5·91	5·86	5·80	5·77	5·75	5·72	5·69	5·66	5·63
5	6·61	5·79	5·41	5·19	5·05	4·95	4·88	4·82	4·77	4·74	4·68	4·62	4·56	4·53	4·50	4·46	4·43	4·40	4·36
6	5·99	5·14	4·76	4·53	4·39	4·28	4·21	4·15	4·10	4·06	4·00	3·94	3·87	3·84	3·81	3·77	3·74	3·70	3·67
7	5·59	4·74	4·35	4·12	3·97	3·87	3·79	3·73	3·68	3·64	3·57	3·51	3·44	3·41	3·38	3·34	3·30	3·27	3·23
8	5·32	4·46	4·07	3·84	3·69	3·58	3·50	3·44	3·39	3·35	3·28	3·22	3·15	3·12	3·08	3·04	3·01	2·97	2·93
9	5·12	4·26	3·86	3·63	3·48	3·37	3·29	3·23	3·18	3·14	3·07	3·01	2·94	2·90	2·86	2·83	2·79	2·75	2·71
10	4·96	4·10	3·71	3·48	3·33	3·22	3·14	3·07	3·02	2·98	2·91	2·85	2·77	2·74	2·70	2·66	2·62	2·58	2·54
11	4·84	3·98	3·59	3·36	3·20	3·09	3·01	2·95	2·90	2·85	2·79	2·72	2·65	2·61	2·57	2·53	2·49	2·45	2·40
12	4·75	3·89	3·49	3·26	3·11	3·00	2·91	2·85	2·80	2·75	2·69	2·62	2·54	2·51	2·47	2·43	2·38	2·34	2·30
13	4·67	3·81	3·41	3·18	3·03	2·92	2·83	2·77	2·71	2·67	2·60	2·53	2·46	2·42	2·38	2·34	2·30	2·25	2·21
14	4·60	3·74	3·34	3·11	2·96	2·85	2·76	2·70	2·65	2·60	2·53	2·46	2·39	2·35	2·31	2·27	2·22	2·18	2·13
15	4·54	3·68	3·29	3·06	2·90	2·79	2·71	2·64	2·59	2·54	2·48	2·40	2·33	2·29	2·25	2·20	2·16	2·11	2·07
16	4·49	3·63	3·24	3·01	2·85	2·74	2·66	2·59	2·54	2·49	2·42	2·35	2·28	2·24	2·19	2·15	2·11	2·06	2·01
17	4·45	3·59	3·20	2·96	2·81	2·70	2·61	2·55	2·49	2·45	2·38	2·31	2·23	2·19	2·15	2·10	2·06	2·01	1·96
18	4·41	3·55	3·16	2·93	2·77	2·66	2·58	2·51	2·46	2·41	2·34	2·27	2·19	2·15	2·11	2·06	2·02	1·97	1·92
19	4·38	3·52	3·13	2·90	2·74	2·63	2·54	2·48	2·42	2·38	2·31	2·23	2·16	2·11	2·07	2·03	1·98	1·93	1·88
20	4·35	3·49	3·10	2·87	2·71	2·60	2·51	2·45	2·39	2·35	2·28	2·20	2·12	2·08	2·04	1·99	1·95	1·90	1·84
21	4·32	3·47	3·07	2·84	2·68	2·57	2·49	2·42	2·37	2·32	2·25	2·18	2·10	2·05	2·01	1·96	1·92	1·87	1·81
22	4·30	3·44	3·05	2·82	2·66	2·55	2·46	2·40	2·34	2·30	2·23	2·15	2·07	2·03	1·98	1·94	1·89	1·84	1·78
23	4·28	3·42	3·03	2·80	2·64	2·53	2·44	2·37	2·32	2·27	2·20	2·13	2·05	2·01	1·96	1·91	1·86	1·81	1·76
24	4·26	3·40	3·01	2·78	2·62	2·51	2·42	2·36	2·30	2·25	2·18	2·11	2·03	1·98	1·94	1·89	1·84	1·79	1·73
25	4·24	3·39	2·99	2·76	2·60	2·49	2·40	2·34	2·28	2·24	2·16	2·09	2·01	1·96	1·92	1·87	1·82	1·77	1·71
26	4·23	3·37	2·98	2·74	2·59	2·47	2·39	2·32	2·27	2·22	2·15	2·07	1·99	1·95	1·90	1·85	1·80	1·75	1·69
27	4·21	3·35	2·96	2·73	2·57	2·46	2·37	2·31	2·25	2·20	2·13	2·06	1·97	1·93	1·88	1·84	1·79	1·73	1·67
28	4·20	3·34	2·95	2·71	2·56	2·45	2·36	2·29	2·24	2·19	2·12	2·04	1·96	1·91	1·87	1·82	1·77	1·71	1·65
29	4·18	3·33	2·93	2·70	2·55	2·43	2·35	2·28	2·22	2·18	2·10	2·03	1·94	1·90	1·85	1·81	1·75	1·70	1·64
30	4·17	3·32	2·92	2·69	2·53	2·42	2·33	2·27	2·21	2·16	2·09	2·01	1·93	1·89	1·84	1·79	1·74	1·68	1·62
40	4·08	3·23	2·84	2·61	2·45	2·34	2·25	2·18	2·12	2·08	2·00	1·92	1·84	1·79	1·74	1·69	1·64	1·58	1·51
60	4·00	3·15	2·76	2·53	2·37	2·25	2·17	2·10	2·04	1·99	1·92	1·84	1·75	1·70	1·65	1·59	1·53	1·47	1·39
120	3·92	3·07	2·68	2·45	2·29	2·17	2·09	2·02	1·96	1·91	1·83	1·75	1·66	1·61	1·55	1·50	1·43	1·35	1·25
∞	3·84	3·00	2·60	2·37	2·21	2·10	2·01	1·94	1·88	1·83	1·75	1·67	1·57	1·52	1·46	1·39	1·32	1·22	1·00

Tables Va and Vb give, respectively, the 95th and 99th percentiles of an F variable with r degrees of freedom in the numerator and s degrees of freedom in the denominator

Table Vb
Upper 1% Points of the F distribution

r / s	1	2	3	4	5	6	7	8	9	10	12	15	20	24	30	40	60	120	∞
1	4052	4999·5	5403	5625	5764	5859	5928	5982	6022	6056	6106	6157	6209	6235	6261	6287	6313	6339	6366
2	98·50	99·00	99·17	99·25	99·30	99·33	99·36	99·37	99·39	99·40	99·42	99·43	99·45	99·46	99·47	99·47	99·48	99·49	99·50
3	34·12	30·82	29·46	28·71	28·24	27·91	27·67	27·49	27·35	27·23	27·05	26·87	26·69	26·60	26·50	26·41	26·32	26·22	26·13
4	21·20	18·00	16·69	15·98	15·52	15·21	14·98	14·80	14·66	14·55	14·37	14·20	14·02	13·93	13·84	13·75	13·65	13·56	13·46
5	16·26	13·27	12·06	11·39	10·97	10·67	10·46	10·29	10·16	10·05	9·89	9·72	9·55	9·47	9·38	9·29	9·20	9·11	9·02
6	13·75	10·92	9·78	9·15	8·75	8·47	8·26	8·10	7·98	7·87	7·72	7·56	7·40	7·31	7·23	7·14	7·06	6·97	6·88
7	12·25	9·55	8·45	7·85	7·46	7·19	6·99	6·84	6·72	6·62	6·47	6·31	6·16	6·07	5·99	5·91	5·82	5·74	5·65
8	11·26	8·65	7·59	7·01	6·63	6·37	6·18	6·03	5·91	5·81	5·67	5·52	5·36	5·28	5·20	5·12	5·03	4·95	4·86
9	10·56	8·02	6·99	6·42	6·06	5·80	5·61	5·47	5·35	5·26	5·11	4·96	4·81	4·73	4·65	4·57	4·48	4·40	4·31
10	10·04	7·56	6·55	5·99	5·64	5·39	5·20	5·06	4·94	4·85	4·71	4·56	4·41	4·33	4·25	4·17	4·08	4·00	3·91
11	9·65	7·21	6·22	5·67	5·32	5·07	4·89	4·74	4·63	4·54	4·40	4·25	4·10	4·02	3·94	3·86	3·78	3·69	3·60
12	9·33	6·93	5·95	5·41	5·06	4·82	4·64	4·50	4·39	4·30	4·16	4·01	3·86	3·78	3·70	3·62	3·54	3·45	3·36
13	9·07	6·70	5·74	5·21	4·86	4·62	4·44	4·30	4·19	4·10	3·96	3·82	3·66	3·59	3·51	3·43	3·34	3·25	3·17
14	8·86	6·51	5·56	5·04	4·69	4·46	4·28	4·14	4·03	3·94	3·80	3·66	3·51	3·43	3·35	3·27	3·18	3·09	3·00
15	8·68	6·36	5·42	4·89	4·56	4·32	4·14	4·00	3·89	3·80	3·67	3·52	3·37	3·29	3·21	3·13	3·05	2·96	2·87
16	8·53	6·23	5·29	4·77	4·44	4·20	4·03	3·89	3·78	3·69	3·55	3·41	3·26	3·18	3·10	3·02	2·93	2·84	2·75
17	8·40	6·11	5·18	4·67	4·34	4·10	3·93	3·79	3·68	3·59	3·46	3·31	3·16	3·08	3·00	2·92	2·83	2·75	2·65
18	8·29	6·01	5·09	4·58	4·25	4·01	3·84	3·71	3·60	3·51	3·37	3·23	3·08	3·00	2·92	2·84	2·75	2·66	2·57
19	8·18	5·93	5·01	4·50	4·17	3·94	3·77	3·63	3·52	3·43	3·30	3·15	3·00	2·92	2·84	2·76	2·67	2·58	2·49
20	8·10	5·85	4·94	4·43	4·10	3·87	3·70	3·56	3·46	3·37	3·23	3·09	2·94	2·86	2·78	2·69	2·61	2·52	2·42
21	8·02	5·78	4·87	4·37	4·04	3·81	3·64	3·51	3·40	3·31	3·17	3·03	2·88	2·80	2·72	2·64	2·55	2·46	2·36
22	7·95	5·72	4·82	4·31	3·99	3·76	3·59	3·45	3·35	3·26	3·12	2·98	2·83	2·75	2·67	2·58	2·50	2·40	2·31
23	7·88	5·66	4·76	4·26	3·94	3·71	3·54	3·41	3·30	3·21	3·07	2·93	2·78	2·70	2·62	2·54	2·45	2·35	2·26
24	7·82	5·61	4·72	4·22	3·90	3·67	3·50	3·36	3·26	3·17	3·03	2·89	2·74	2·66	2·58	2·49	2·40	2·31	2·21
25	7·77	5·57	4·68	4·18	3·85	3·63	3·46	3·32	3·22	3·13	2·99	2·85	2·70	2·62	2·54	2·45	2·36	2·27	2·17
26	7·72	5·53	4·64	4·14	3·82	3·59	3·42	3·29	3·18	3·09	2·96	2·81	2·66	2·58	2·50	2·42	2·33	2·23	2·13
27	7·68	5·49	4·60	4·11	3·78	3·56	3·39	3·26	3·15	3·06	2·93	2·78	2·63	2·55	2·47	2·38	2·29	2·20	2·10
28	7·64	5·45	4·57	4·07	3·75	3·53	3·36	3·23	3·12	3·03	2·90	2·75	2·60	2·52	2·44	2·35	2·26	2·17	2·06
29	7·60	5·42	4·54	4·04	3·73	3·50	3·33	3·20	3·09	3·00	2·87	2·73	2·57	2·49	2·41	2·33	2·23	2·14	2·03
30	7·56	5·39	4·51	4·02	3·70	3·47	3·30	3·17	3·07	2·98	2·84	2·70	2·55	2·47	2·39	2·30	2·21	2·11	2·01
40	7·31	5·18	4·31	3·83	3·51	3·29	3·12	2·99	2·89	2·80	2·66	2·52	2·37	2·29	2·20	2·11	2·02	1·92	1·80
60	7·08	4·98	4·13	3·65	3·34	3·12	2·95	2·82	2·72	2·63	2·50	2·35	2·20	2·12	2·03	1·94	1·84	1·73	1·60
120	6·85	4·79	3·95	3·48	3·17	2·96	2·79	2·66	2·56	2·47	2·34	2·19	2·03	1·95	1·86	1·76	1·66	1·53	1·38
∞	6·63	4·61	3·78	3·32	3·02	2·80	2·64	2·51	2·41	2·32	2·18	2·04	1·88	1·79	1·70	1·59	1·47	1·32	1·00

SOME FREQUENTLY USED SYMBOLS

μ	the mean of a population
σ	the standard deviation of a population
p	the proportion in a population
N	size of population
n	size of sample
$\overline{X}$	the variable representing the mean of a sample
$\overline{x}$	the numerical value of the mean of a sample
s	the standard deviation of a sample
H_0	the null hypothesis
P( )	probability of the event enclosed between parentheses
S.E.( )	Standard error of the statistic enclosed between parentheses
d.f.	degrees of freedom
$z(\alpha)$	the value of a standard normal variable which is exceeded with probability α
$t_r(\alpha)$	the value of a t variable (with r degrees of freedom) which is exceeded with probability α
$\chi_r^2(\alpha)$	the value of a Chi-square variable (with r degrees of freedom) which is exceeded with probability α
$F_{m,n}(\alpha)$	the value of an F variable (with m degrees of freedom in its numerator and n in its denominator) which is exceeded with probability α

Index